LIBR A

Also by Sally Glen (with Maggie Nicol):

Clinical Skills in Nursing: The Return of the Practical Room?
(Macmillan, 1999)

Problem-based Learning in Nursing

A new model for a new context?

Edited by

Sally Glen

and

Kay Wilkie

First published 2000 by
MACMILLAN PRESS LTD
Houndmills, Basingstoke, Hampshire RG21 6XS
and London
Companies and representatives throughout the world

ISBN 0–333–77014–5 paperback

A catalogue record for this book is available from the British Library.

This book is printed on paper suitable for recycling and made from fully managed and sustained forest sources.

10   9   8   7   6   5   4   3   2   1
09 08 07 06 05 04 03 02 01 00

Editing and origination by
Aardvark Editorial, Mendham, Suffolk

Printed in Malaysia

Contents

List of Figures and Tables

Figures

Tables

List of Contributors

Iain Burns Programme Leader, Adult Branch, School of Nursing and Midwifery, University of Dundee.

Sally Glen Professor of Nursing Education and Dean, St Bartholomew's School of Nursing and Midwifery, City University.

Carolyn Gibbon Senior Lecturer, School of Health, Liverpool John Moores University.

Sue Grandis Enquiry-based Learning Project Co-ordinator, School of Nursing and Midwifery, University of Southampton.

Garth Long formerly Director of Pre-Registration Studies, School of Nursing and Midwifery, University of Southampton, now Professional Officer, English National Board.

Di Marks-Maran Head of Centre for Teaching and Learning, Wolfson School of Health Sciences, Thames Valley University.

Bob Price Distance Learning Programme Director, The RCN Institute, London.

Maggi Savin-Baden Principal Lecturer, School of Health and Social Science, University of Coventry.

B. Gail Thomas Dean of Midwifery and Child Health, Wolfson School of Health Sciences, Thames Valley University.

Kay Wilkie PBL Co-ordinator, School of Nursing and Midwifery, University of Dundee.

Joyce Wise Senior Lecturer, School of Nursing and Midwifery, University of Portsmouth.

Foreword

Why a new model for a new context? Although problem-based learning has been around for some time, having been pioneered in medicine and then taken up in such disciplines as architecture, dentistry, biology, physiotherapy and journalism, it is comparatively new to nursing. By changing the focus on learning from a subject-based to a more problem-focused curriculum it represents a qualitative shift in pedagogical philosophy and practice. It emphasises co-operation rather than competition, and small-group learning rather than teacher-focused teaching. Problem-based learning encourages the deep learning that occurs when students actively engage in their own discovery, and when they are given the opportunity to choose their preferred methods of research.

Problem-based learning works by presenting students with a problem and then allowing them to research it in a safe environment. It does not provide lectures, but rather supports the students with resources in order for them to discover what they need to know. Learning occurs in groups so that students can support each other, but also because nurses work this way in the workplaces, and must discover ways of doing so effectively.

Problem-based learning is in the ascendancy in nurse education; it is being taken up enthusiastically in schools and faculties of nursing around the world in places as diverse as South East Asia, Japan, Turkey, Australia, Canada and the United Kingdom. Nurses have recognised that it is no longer enough to obey orders unthinkingly, nor to rely on knowledge which is out of date almost as soon as it is taught. Wherever I present workshops on problem-based learning I see a desire to have students think critically for themselves and to have them work as active partners in the learning process.

This represents a huge change for us as teachers. It means that we must think differently about our roles, that we must be facilitators of student learning, that we must structure the curriculum so that students can work systematically through a body of knowledge that they must possess, and that we must be more creative in devising assessment that will support problem-based learning. It means that we must research what we do. We must make sure that this new (and infinitely more enjoyable) way of teaching, does not suffer from a 'halo' effect, but is shown to be more effective in helping students learn, and to continue to learn long after they have left the university.

It also represents a new role for students, who need to understand from the very beginning of a programme of study what we are trying to achieve together. They must learn that we value what they bring from their life experience, and that they will learn best if they take an active part in that learning. It may take some time for students who have been used to a more didactic form of learning to believe us when we say we value what they do both individually and in groups. The ways we can convince them will be by effective facilitation, by well-structured curricula and well-presented learning materials, and by designing assessment which challenges them to think critically rather than to reproduce material in a rote fashion.

Problem-based learning is an effective way of teaching and learning in nursing because its processes mimic those used in the clinical reasoning process on which nursing is based. Students can apprehend clinical problems, can hypothesise about them and can, on the basis of those hypotheses, make clinical judgements. In turn such judgements will guide nursing care and provide for its evaluation. As Francis Biley and Keri Smith suggest in their 1998 paper 'The Buck Stops Here', students of problem-based programmes think about what they do before they do it, reflect on what they have done in order to improve future performance, and take responsibility for their actions in relation to learning and in offering nursing care.

'Problem-Based Learning in Nursing: A New Model for a New Context?' aims to 'offer ideas, practical advice and guidance to those developing problem-based learning in nursing and midwifery curricula'. It achieves this admirably in offering snapshots of successful implementation at nursing and midwifery schools in the United Kingdom. There is much here to help those who want to set up programmes, or parts of programmes, using problem-based learning. As well there is a real engagement with the philosophy of problem-based learning: an examination of the things that work and those which don't. There is a sustained engagement here with teaching and nursing, and the ways in which we can most effectively prepare nurses for the next millennium.

Nursing is now firmly grounded in universities. This gives us the opportunity to provide students with freedoms they have not formerly possessed to find and use knowledge in ways which will enrich their practice. Employers want nurses to be able to respond quickly and appropriately to patients' needs. Students want to feel confident and part of nursing culture and want to make changes to the ways in which nursing is practised. This book foregrounds those concerns, and suggests ways in which nurses will be equipped to deal with them. It takes forward the debate on problem-based learning in nursing in both theoretical and practical ways. It is a timely and useful contribution. One which does indeed offer alternatives for a new context but which will, in turn, change the context in which we can practise as nurses.

CHRISTINE ALAVI
Griffith University, Queensland, Australia

Preface

The aim of this book is to offer ideas, practical advice and guidance to those developing and implementing problem-based learning (PBL) in nursing and midwifery curricula.

Chapter 1 contextualises the recent development of PBL in nursing and midwifery education. Nursing and midwifery educationalists have a responsibility to encourage and develop creative, critical thinkers who can respond to the rapidly changing healthcare environment and the requirements of demanding healthcare consumers. This requires the identification of opportunities for students to develop transferable skills such as problem-solving, critical thinking and the ability to work independently and in groups. There is thus an increasing emphasis on ensuring that nurses and midwives are self-reliant, efficient professionals who are capable of researching and examining problems within the workplace. There also appears to be a widespread view that university educators in general may need to focus more on activities that relate learning to professional life in the practice area. One response to this challenge has been the development of learning experiences based upon the principles of PBL.

Chapter 2 explores definitions and models of PBL, its strengths and limitations as a technique and its potential application to nursing and midwifery education. PBL is the subject of much controversy, partly as a result of misapplications and misapprehensions about its use. PBL can have many different meanings, depending on the design of the educational method employed and the skills of the lecturer. Educators should be aware that different educational objectives can be achieved by different approaches. Care should also be taken in implementing PBL to ensure that the intended outcomes will be achieved. PBL is much more than a simple teaching strategy. It is a technique that offers nursing and midwifery students the opportunity to adopt a deep learning approach to identifying problematic issues, recognising individual learning needs, organising themselves to acquire the knowledge and applying it to the situation. PBL also takes hard work and commitment at all levels – it cannot be regarded as a 'quick fix'. However, PBL has the potential to respond rapidly to changes in professional knowledge and to promote evidence-based practice and team-working – all valuable attributes for a career as a qualified nurse or midwife.

Chapter 3 describes the process of introducing PBL into a preregistration programme. The chapter focuses particularly on practical issues, such as the identification of resources (human and material) and staff development. A staff development strategy is described that focuses on facilitation, informing and preparing clinical staff, and developing learning materials. Other practical issues, such as the need to reflect the PBL process in the assessment, are also discussed. Finally, the importance of evaluation is noted. This issue of assessment and evaluation within the context of PBL is further developed in Chapter 8.

Chapter 4 describes the introduction of an enquiry-based learning (EBL) whole-programme approach in preregistration/ undergraduate nursing and midwifery. This chapter suggests that the term 'enquiry-based learning' captures students' initial motivation and the continuing need for individuals to learn, to seek stimulation to learn, and to be permitted to explore the status of current knowledge on a wide range of issues relevant to health. EBL is complemented by the notion of evidence-based practice, with the ever-present need to review the rationale for assumed knowledge. A whole-programme integrated approach is achieved by presenting the learning content in scenarios to provide the initial stimulus to motivate broad and deep learning. Chapter 4 emphasises the need to ensure that everyone involved in programme delivery understands the philosophy of EBL, supports it, owns it and develops it further. Support from the 'top' is also cited as being important, in addition to keeping lecturers informed, listening and giving credit, and a related staff development programme.

Chapter 5 outlines how a maternity service in England responded to the Winterton report, particularly, how a close working relationship between clinical and education colleagues helped to prepare midwives who are competent and confident to implement a case-holding style of service delivery. An educational strategy was needed that was flexible enough to take into account the multiplicity of midwives' backgrounds and experience, but focused enough to ensure that the learning achieved was relevant to the needs of each midwife. The education strategy also needed to be manageable practically in terms of structure and delivery, as well as financially. The starting point in addressing this issue was to consider exactly what was required in practical terms. In essence, midwives needed to direct their own learning in a way that mirrored the work pattern they would be required to adopt. A form of open/distance learning seemed to be the most obvious and flexible solution. An adult learning approach was considered essential, and a PBL component was eventually developed as an integral feature. However, it must be stressed that it was essential to work *with* the midwives on this project rather than to offer an imposed strategy. In this way, a sense of ownership could develop that was likely to increase its chance of success.

Chapter 6 examines the extent to which the groups in which students work and learn are effective. All too often, PBL is implemented with little attention being paid to the relative costs and benefits of group-based learning. This chapter explores the importance of acknowledging that students participating in PBL work in teams rather than groups. The notion of interactional stance is also examined. Research into PBL demonstrates that staff and students' ability to work and learn effectively within teams is affected by the position they choose to take up within a PBL team: their interactional stance. The concept of disjunction is also explored; this can be defined as becoming completely 'stuck' in learning, as feeling fragmented. The result is frustration, confusion and often a demand for the 'right' answers. The effective management of disjunction will mean not only that students will develop generally applicable competences, but also that they will be able to adapt them and critique their value throughout their professional lives. Change is then seen as a feature of their professional lives rather than a fault. Finally, critique becomes the touchstone of professional self-management.

Chapter 7 explores the possible benefit of combining PBL and distance learning in order to enrich the education of nurses and midwives. To do this, it is necessary to question the tenets of distance learning within the UK. What has been fundamentally flawed within a classical model of distance learning is an unclear, often inadequate, utilisation of the tutor-counsellor and a belief that learning materials, however well written, should be directed towards teaching rather than the facilitation of learning.

Chapter 7 suggests that PBL within a distance learning programme is both possible and, indeed, desirable, but a number of issues require careful attention. For example, one needs to consider whether PBL should be the sole philosophy underpinning a curriculum, or whether it in fact represents a complementary approach to more traditional, perhaps deductive, learning within nurse education. In addition to the philosophical questions, the case study presented in Chapter 8 raises issues related to the preparation of material and support services within distance learning. Just as distance learning serves to highlight some of the opportunities and limitations associated with PBL, so PBL enables one to question some of the treasured assumptions about distance learning. Irrespective of whether PBL becomes a prominent feature within distance learning education curricula, its lessons should be understood with regard to writing of distance learning materials and the organisation of tutor-counsellor support.

Chapter 8 explores two issues that are fundamental to PBL programmes: assessment and evaluation. Because the terms 'assessment' and 'evaluation' mean different things to different people, the chapter begins by offering definitions of these two educational terms. PBL presents unique challenges with regard to the assessment of student achievement and the evaluation of the programme. There is also an imperative within PBL to obtain evaluation data in order to make evidence-based decisions concerning programme development. The literature offers a wide range of assessment and evaluation methods that are compatible and congruent with PBL. The primary principle remaining, however, is that when PBL is introduced the assessment techniques and evaluation methods must reflect the underlying principles and intentions of PBL.

Chapter 9 concludes by suggesting that modern nursing is still evolving. Just as nursing practice adapts to changes in healthcare provision, so must nurse education if it is to remain current. If nurses are to be prepared for a pivotal role in the care of people in the twenty-first century, nurse education has to develop innovative and creative initiatives to meet the needs of the citizens of the region served. Nurse educationalists thus have a responsibility to encourage and develop nurses who can respond proactively to the rapidly changing healthcare environment and the requirements of demanding healthcare consumers. This chapter suggests that, to meet this challenge, nurse education must pass two basic tests. The first is how well it equips nurses to apply their knowledge in contexts beyond the bounds of their formal educational experience, and the second, how well it motivates and equips nurses to continue learning throughout their professional lives. The passing of these two basic tests may require a new model of nurse education. PBL curricula could provide the framework for the revolution in nursing education to occur. In essence, it could provide a new model of nursing education.

SALLY GLEN
City University
KAY WILKIE
University of Dundee

Acknowledgements

The editors wish to thank all the contributors for helping to further the debate on problem-based learning in professional education. We would also like to thank Janice Duffy for her administrative and secretarial support.

Every effort has been made to trace all the copyright holders but if any have been inadvertently overlooked the publishers will be pleased to make the necessary arrangements at the first opportunity.

1

A New Model for a New Context?

Iain Burns and Sally Glen

Introduction

A framework known as Project 2000 was established in 1986 for nursing and midwifery education and practice. Historically, views on how best to prepare nurses and midwives have reflected existing ideologies in both education and nursing, which have in turn reflected the prevailing social climate (Spouse, 1998). Project 2000's intentions were to produce nurses and midwives better able to meet the rapidly changing healthcare needs of society. A framework was thus established that produced not just safe nurses and midwives, but nurses and midwives who were able to improve the quality of patient care and were 'fit for purpose' (UKCC, 1986). The question of whether student nurses and midwives are prepared to meet the demands of clinical practice at the point of registration has been debated under the heading 'fitness for purpose'. A fundamental principle of preregistration nursing and midwifery education, since the establishment of the Project 2000 framework, is the extent to which it provides new practitioners with an appropriate foundation for practice (Luker *et al.*, 1996). There are growing concerns about whether education programmes are equipping nurses with the necessary knowledge and skills base for accountable practice (Scott, 1997; Walsh, 1997; Runciman *et al.*, 1998; DoH, 1999; UKCC, 1999). However, May *et al.* (1997), while recognising the need for a continual evalua-

1

tion of the Project 2000 programmes introduced in Scotland in 1992, indicated that the profession 'seems to be on the right track in our preparation of tomorrow's practitioners'.

Replacement of the traditional training model

The first Diploma of Nursing and Midwifery in Higher Education (DipHE) programmes commenced in September 1989. Until 1989, Registered General Nurse programmes were based on apprentice-type models, with much reliance upon experience gained in the clinical setting (traditionally the hospital) as a means of acquiring knowledge and skills. Traditional nurse education has been described and characterised by rigidly prescribed nursing curricula, preconceived ideas about the way in which students learn and should be taught, and the repression of creativity (de Tornyay, 1990). In adopting this type of approach, it has been suggested that nurses, once qualified, fail to exhibit patient-oriented critical thinking and are not capable of adequate decision-making in practice (Heliker, 1994). The move of educational programmes from monotechnic and National Health Service (NHS) managed settings to Institutes of Higher Education heralded the demise of traditional training programmes centred in hospital Colleges of Nursing and Midwifery. The introduction of the DipHE in 1989 meant that programmes of education offered students professional registration, but also for the first time located nursing and midwifery education completely within the higher education system. These reforms thus led to the replacement of the traditional training models (Glen, 1999).

The diploma structure brought with it an increased emphasis on health promotion and the prevention of illness. There has also been a dramatic increase in the time spent studying subjects such as psychology, sociology and health policy. One of the issues that has emerged from Fitness for Practice (UKCC, 1999) is an overemphasis on academic achievement to the detriment of practice experience. The emphasis placed on the theoretical elements of the programmes, and the significant reduction in the time that students spend on acquiring psychomotor skills in the university (Luker *et al.*, 1996; Runciman *et al.*, 1998), has resulted in the curriculum becoming overloaded, encouraging the development of surface as opposed to deeper learning (Margetson, 1994). Some believe that current preregistration education may have too much theory and too little practice, particularly in the early stages (Hislop *et al.*, 1996). It could also be argued that there is insufficient attention to the integration of theory and practice in the real world. This has led to the inclusion of inappropriate or irrelevant material within the curriculum.

It is not surprising that Scott (1997, p. 5) reported that, in many instances, students were 'not prepared for the work they have to do'. The location of nursing and midwifery education in higher education has thus led to the diminution of learning by doing, as in apprenticeship training, and a corresponding increase in theory-led curricula. There appears to be a widespread view that educators and the university sector in general may need to focus more on activities that relate learning to life in the practice area (Hilton, 1992). May *et al.* (1997) noted that the introduction of Project 2000 also introduced 'radical concepts' such as student-centred pedagogy, the integration of theory and practice, reflective learning and lifelong learning.

Lifelong learning

The traditional pattern of nursing and midwifery education, which relied heavily on teaching factual knowledge, and a demand for lecturers to cover all possible content (Ryan, 1993), did not foster independent learning, critical reasoning or problem-solving. This encouraged students to concentrate on knowledge-gathering as an end in itself rather than on the knowledge needed for practice (Sadlo *et al.*, 1994). This approach had become inadequate and outmoded by the early 1980s (Studdy *et al.*, 1994). Recent developments in medical technology and practices, as well as changes in the social climate, have increased patients' expectations and radically altered the nature of nursing practice. The advent of 'new nursing' (Beardshaw and Robinson, 1990), requiring collaborative patient care and sophisticated nursing knowledge and techniques, places greater and explicit burdens of accountability and responsibility on professional staff. As a result, practitioners have to reconceptualise their practice using research-based evidence to support their decisions. Nursing is consequently becoming increasingly sophisticated, with a low centralisation of decision-making processes.

Learning itself is now regarded as a lifelong activity, not something sandwiched between childhood and work. The Dearing and Garrick reports (National Committee of Enquiry into Higher Education, 1997a, 1997b) and the White Paper *The Learning Age* (DfEE, 1998) emphasise the utilisation of flexible, self-directed approaches in preference to more traditional methods of teaching and learning, which are more teacher centred in approach. There is an assumption that nursing and midwifery education should provide students with a variety of learning experiences and hence transferable skills. Transferable skills include problem-solving, verbal communication, self-enquiry, self-confidence, self-discipline and team-working. The inability to work easily with other people as a member of a team is consistently identified by employers as a deficit (Levin, 1998).

Students need to be facilitated to become more responsible for their own learning and be given the experience to acquire the appropriate skills to support this. The purpose of getting students to participate in these kinds of activity is to encourage self-reliance, self-regulation and self-directed learning (Knowles, 1990). Collaborative and peer learning activities, participatory, interactive learning and interdisciplinary learning are increasingly cited as models of good nursing and midwifery educational practice (Hickie, 1998). The key issue seems to be that students need to be encouraged and motivated to learn and know how to learn if they are to develop lifelong learning skills (Amos and White, 1998). In addition, nurses and midwives need to be exposed to opportunities in which they not only learn how to learn, but also enjoy the learning experience enough to continue learning throughout life.

The skills of lifelong learning include the ability to identify a need, access and retrieve information, filter it for quality in relation to a specific client/patient problem and then use the information to provide the most appropriate care required. Equipped with these skills, novice nurses and midwives are prepared for flexible, professional learning and development in a multidisciplinary, multisite health service in the twenty-first century.

Schools and departments of nursing and midwifery now aim to provide academic and professional programmes to meet the lifetime learning needs of their students, graduates and health-care providers by developing portfolios of flexible continuing professional development and distance learning programmes to meet the needs of professional bodies and employers, and by the accreditation of prior learning and the mainstreaming of work-based and problem-based learning. They also encourage students to take a more active responsibility for their own learning experience. Students are encouraged to become increasingly responsible for their own work and the acquisition of appropriate skills to support their studies. The purpose of getting students to participate in these types of activity is to encourage self-reliance and self-regulation.

The clinical environment is not designed for the task of learning in practice: it is a setting designed for the care of patients in which practice necessarily dominates (Hewison and Wildman, 1996). Far-reaching changes in both healthcare needs and service provision also make it increasingly difficult for student nurses and midwives to develop skills through repetition (Runciman *et al.*, 1998; Glen, 1999). These changes include a decline in the number of acute hospital beds, an increased emphasis on day surgery and a move towards home care, coupled with a major shift of resources into primary healthcare provision. Patients are also often more sick and should not be subjected to the practice of the complete novice (Studdy *et al.*, 1994). Students now spend less time in the hospital ward setting, where nurses and midwives have traditionally developed and practised their nursing and midwifery skills and knowledge. Placements have also become an increasingly specialised, often unpredictable, resource (May *et al.*, 1997).

While the primary and formal responsibility for the education of nursing students rests with the education institution, it also depends significantly on effective teaching support, and on supervision and assessment by preceptors, assessors and mentors in clinical areas, for whom this is an additional role amounting to work overload (Barrett and Myrick, 1998). The NHS reforms have resulted in clinical staff having to balance conflicting demands in their management, clinical and education roles (Jowett *et al.*, 1994). In addition, the labour intensity of health-care (Buchan, 1994), as well as the promotion of the most clinically skilled staff, has served to militate against clinical staff's ability to achieve 'fitness for purpose'. Clinical staff have also

expressed concern about: finding enough qualified staff to act
as supervisors; the learning burden of supervision given student
and staff numbers; and the heightened demands in terms of
time and responsibility of teaching and supervising students
undertaking the Common Foundation Programme (CFP), who
possess not even basic practical nursing skills (Bedford *et al.*, 1993;
Elkan and Robinson, 1995). May *et al.* (1997) also noted that
the availability of mentors in the placement area was limited. Similarly, the respondents in Luker *et al.*'s (1996) study were keen
to acknowledge their responsibilities with regard to providing
an optimum clinical learning environment for students. The
reality for them was of working in a context that did not support
this aim. Concurrently, the higher education system has also
radically changed in the past 15 years.

Changes in the higher education system

Since the mid-1980s, the UK's higher education system has taken
on a different meaning from its previous rather exclusive conno-
tations. The millennium makes bold headlines with slogans about
'access', the 'learning society' and 'lifelong learning'. The channels of access to higher education have been broadened and
multiplied. The profile of the student nurse and midwife population has been transformed, which in effect means that nursing
has to 'address a wider range of abilities, age, background and
motivation for entry than any other discipline' (Creedy and
Alavi, 1997, p. 219). The expectation and learning styles of
students are also increasingly diverse (Cavanagh *et al.*, 1994).

If a system is to make itself accessible and attractive to a much
wider and more varied section of the population than hitherto,
it seems inescapable that there will need to be a movement away
from disciplinary specialisation within higher education. Much of
the learning within the higher education section can become 'academic' and of little relevance to the 'real world' of the practice
setting (Schön, 1983). The induction into the discipline approach
contributes little to the development of skills of issue clarification
and problem formulation in areas that do not fall immediately
within the remit of the given discipline, issues of the very type
that nursing and midwifery students are likely to confront outside

discipline boundaries in the world of practice (Glen, 1995). Qualified nurses or midwives may be limited in their ability to apply theoretical knowledge to the clinical situation. Support for the notion that theory derived within discipline-based enquiry can be directly applied to practice has dwindled over the last two decades (Hirst, 1979; McIntyre, 1980; Tom, 1980); instead, it has increasingly been recognised that learning knowledge and using knowledge are not separate processes but the same process (Eraut, 1994). Everyday human learning is a context-dependent and socially mediated activity. Learning to be a nurse or midwife is thus a more complex and problematic activity than the literature would lead us to believe (Spouse, 1998).

Conclusion

With the advent of Project 2000, it was recognised that if the profession were to meet its target of educating practitioners capable of responding flexibly and critically to changing healthcare needs of patients, clients and society at large, a different approach to professional development was needed. Healthcare organisations are now seeking a responsive, adaptable workforce who are prepared to be lifelong learners, adapting and changing as required by the organisation.

Nursing and midwifery educationalists have a responsibility to encourage and develop creative, critical thinkers who can respond to the rapidly changing healthcare environment and the requirements of demanding healthcare consumers. This requires the identification of opportunities for students to develop transferable skills such as problem-solving, critical thinking and the ability to work independently and in groups. There is an increasing emphasis on ensuring that nurses and midwives are self-reliant, efficient professionals who are capable of researching and examining problems within the workplace.

Problem-based learning (PBL) is offered by many as a solution to some of the problems within professional education, and is considered to have several advantages over more traditional methods of education. First, student motivation tends to be high because the material presented is relevant and applicable to the clinical situation. Second, the emphasis is on encouraging the students to use their existing knowledge, a deficiency of traditional passive teaching methods (Amos and White, 1998), and to explore 'what needs to be known to address and improve a particular situation' (Boud and Feletti, 1997, p. 16). Finally, Alavi (1995) suggests that it allows the integration of theory and practice through the use of real problem situations within the curriculum. Thus, knowledge will be retained in a manner that is applicable to practice, rather than on a purely intellectual basis, and will be reinforced by dealing with similar problems within the clinical environment. The aim is to improve problem-solving skills and relate theoretical principles to clinical reality. In adopting this approach, students also accept the primary responsibility for their own learning and become fully involved in the learning process (Doring *et al.*, 1995). The skills that are developed through this process are intended to facilitate life-long learning and the ability to deal with problematic situations encountered during their professional lives.

References

Alavi, C (1995) Introduction. In Alavi, C (ed.) *Problem-based Learning in a Health Sciences Curriculum*, London: Routledge.

Amos, E and White, M J (1998) Teaching Tools: Problem-based Learning, *Nurse Educator*, **23**(2): 11–14.

Barrett, C and Myrick, F (1998) Job Satisfaction in Preceptorship and its Effect on the Clinical Performance of the Preceptor, *Journal of Advanced Nursing*, **27**: 364–7.

Beardshaw, V and Robinson R (1990) *New for Old? Projects for Nursing in the 1990s*, Research Report No. 8, London: King's Fund Institute.

Bedford, H, Phillips, T, Robinson, J and Shostak, J (1993) *Assessing Competencies in Nursing and Midwifery Education*, London: ENB.

Boud, D and Feletti, G (1997) Changing Problem-based Learning. Introduction. In Boud, D and Feletti, G (eds) *The Challenge of Problem-based Learning* (2nd edn), London: Kogan Page.

Buchan, J (1994) Nursing Shortages and Human Resource Planning, *International Journal of Nursing Studies*, **31**(5): 460–70.

Cavanagh, S J, Hogan, K and Ramgopal, T (1994) Student Nurse Learning Styles, *Senior Nurse*, **13**(7): 37–41.

Creedy, D and Alavi, C (1997) Problem-based Learning in an Integrated Nursing Curriculum. In Boud, D and Feletti, G (eds), *The Challenge of Problem-based Learning*, London: Kogan Page.

Department for Education and Employment (1998) *The Learning Age: A Renaissance for a New Britain,* London: HMSO.

Department of Health (1999) *Making a Difference: Strengthening the Nursing, Midwifery and Health Visiting Contribution to Health and Healthcare,* London: Stationery Office.

Doring, A, Bramwell, A and Bingham, B (1995) Staff Comfort/ Discomfort with Problem-based Learning: A Preliminary Study, *Nurse Education Today,* **15**(4): 263–6.

Elkan, R and Robinson, J (1995) Project 2000: A Review of Published Research, *Journal of Advanced Nursing,* **22**: 386–92.

Eraut, M (1994) *Developing Professional Knowledge and Competence,* London: Falmer Press.

Glen, S (1995) Towards a New Model of Nursing Education, *Nurse Education Today,* **15**: 90–5.

Glen, S (1999) The Demise of the Apprenticeship Model. In Nicol, M and Glen, S (eds), *Clinical Skills in Nursing: Return of the Practical Room?,* Basingstoke: Macmillan.

Heliker, D (1994) Meeting the Challenge of the Curriculum Revolution: Problem-based Learning in Nurse Education, *Journal of Nursing Education,* **33**: 45–7.

Hewison, A and Wildman, S (1996) The Theory–Practice Gap in Nursing: A New Dimension, *Journal of Advanced Nursing,* **24**: 754–61.

Hickie, S (1998) *Information Base on Arrangements which Support the Development of Clinical Practice in Pre-registration Nursing Programmes in Scotland,* Edinburgh: NBS.

Hilton, P (1992) Clinical Skills Laboratories: Teaching Practice Nursing, *Nursing Standard,* **10**(37): 44–7.

Hirst, P H (1979) Professional Studies in Initial Teacher Education: Some Conceptual Issues. In Alexander, R J and Wormald, E (eds) *Professional Studies for Teaching,* Guildford: Society for Research in Higher Education.

Hislop, S, Inglis, B, Cope, P, Stoddart, B and McIntosh, C (1996) Situating Theory in Practice: Student Views of Theory and Practice in Project 2000 Nursing Programmes, *Journal of Advanced Nursing,* **23**: 171–7.

Jowett, S, Walton, I and Payne, S (1994) *Challenges and Changes in Nurse Education – Study of the Implementation of Project 2000,* Slough: National Foundation for Educational Research in England and Wales.

Knowles, M (1990) *The Adult Learner: The Neglected Species,* Houston: Gulf.

Levin, P (1998) Divided they Surely Fall, *Times Higher,* 6 February, p. 28.

Luker, K, Carlisle, C, Riley, E, Stilwell, B, Davies, C and Wilson, R (1996) *Project 2000 Fitness for Purpose: Report to the Department of Health,* University of Liverpool and University of Warwick.

McIntyre, D (1980) The Contribution of Research to Quality in Teacher Education. In Hoyle, E and Megarry, J (eds) *Professional Development of Teachers, World Yearbook of Education*, London: Kogan Page.

Margetson, D (1994) Current Educational Reform and the Significance of Problem-based Learning, *Studies in Higher Education*, **19**(1): 5–19.

May, N, Vetch, L, McIntosh, J and Alexander, M (1997) *Preparation for Practice: Evaluation of Nurse and Midwife Education in Scotland, 1992 Programmes, Final Report*, Edinburgh: NBS.

National Committee of Enquiry into Higher Education, (Chairman R Dearing) (1997a) *Higher Education in the Learning Society*, London: NCIHE.

National Committee of Enquiry into Higher Education, (Chairman R Garrick, Scottish Committee) (1997b) *Higher Education in the Learning Society: Report of the Scottish Committee*, Edinburgh: NCIHE.

Runciman P, Dewar B and Goulbourne A (1998) *Employers' Needs and the Skills of Newly Qualified Project 2000 Staff Nurses*, Edinburgh: Queen Margaret College.

Ryan, G (1993) Student Perceptions about Self-directed Learning in a Professional Course Implementing Problem-based Learning, *Studies in Higher Education*, **18**(1): 53–63.

Sadlo, G, Waren Piper, D and Agnew, P (1994) Problem-based Learning in the Development of an Occupational Therapy Curriculum, Part 1: The Process of Problem-based Learning, *British Journal of Occupational Therapy*, **57**(2): 49–54.

Schön, D A (1983) *The Reflective Practitioner: How Professionals Think in Action*, Aldershot: Arena.

Scott, G (1997) Diploma Nurses Need Extra Year to Gain Clinical Skills, *Nursing Standard*, **12**(1): 5.

Spouse, J (1998) Learning to Nurse through Legitimate Peripheral Participation, *Nurse Education Today* **18**: 345–51.

Studdy, S J, Nicol, M and Fox-Hiley, A (1994) Teaching and Learning Clinical Skills Part of Development of a Teaching Model and Schedule of Skills Development, *Nurse Education Today*, **14**: 186–93.

Tom, A (1980) The Reform of Teacher Education through Research: A Futile Quest, *Teachers College Record*, **82**(1): 15–29.

Tornyay, R de (1990) The Curriculum Revolution, *Journal of Nursing Education*, **29**: 292–4.

United Kingdom Central Council for Nursing, Midwifery and Health Visiting (1986) *Project 2000: A New Preparation for Practice*, London: UKCC.

United Kingdom Central Council for Nursing, Midwifery and Health Visiting (1999) *Fitness for Practice*, London: UKCC.

Walsh, M (1997) Accountability and Intuition: Justifying Nursing Practice, *Nursing Standard*, **11**(23): 39–41.

2

The Nature of Problem-based Learning

Kay Wilkie

Defining PBL

> No doubt, problem-based learning is the basic human learning process
> that allowed primitive man to survive in his environment. (Barrows
> and Tamblyn, 1980, p. 72)

PBL is an instructional method in which students work in small
groups to gain knowledge and acquire problem-solving skills. A
major characteristic of PBL is that the problem is presented to
the students *before* the material has been learned rather than
after, as in the more traditional 'problem-solving approach'. A
second notable feature of PBL is that the problems are presented
in the context in which students are likely to encounter the
given (or a similar) problem in real life. It is this contextualisation of material which makes PBL an attractive strategy for
the education of professionals (cf. Chapter 1).

Howard Barrows, regarded by many as one of PBL's founding
fathers, wrote in 1986 of PBL as a reiterative or 'closed loop' process
of 'encountering the problem first, problem-solving with clinical
reasoning skill and identifying learning needs, self-study, applying
newly gained knowledge to the problem and summarising what
has been learned'. Although attractive, PBL is also the subject of
much controversy, partly as a result of misapplications and misapprehensions concerning its use (Boud and Feletti, 1997).

Barrows (1986) states that 'problem-based learning' can have many different meanings depending on the design of the educational method employed and the skills of the lecturer. Educators may be unaware that different educational objectives can be achieved by the different approaches. Care should be taken in implementing PBL to ensure that the intended outcomes will be achieved.

The 'problem' in the title 'problem-based learning' is itself problematic. Many lecturers dislike the implication that either the patient or learning need is a 'problem', that something has gone wrong and requires to be fixed. Many patient/client or student issues that require a response are not 'problems' but are, conversely, interventions that are undertaken to prevent problems. This view has led to some PBL courses being entitled 'enquiry/inquiry-based learning (E/IBL) or task-based learning (TBL). As both these strategies have attributes that are similar to, but different from, PBL, determining the actual nature of a course can be confusing. The term 'based' also gives rise to discussion. Margetson (1994) suggests that the problem is not the *base* for the learning, but the item that is used to focus the learning. The term 'problem-focused learning' is more accurate, but as PBL is the standard term, its use continues. PBL has also developed its own terminology, for example 'triggers' and 'SIPS', which may vary slightly from one organisation to another. A glossary of some of the terms is given at the end of the chapter.

PBL encourages open-minded, reflective, critical and active learning; it acknowledges that both teachers and students have knowledge, understanding, feelings and a shared interest in the educational process. It also reflects the complex and ever-changing nature of knowledge and the need for learning to continue throughout life. Knowing 'that' is insufficient: we also need to know 'how'. The effect of situation, experience and culture on knowledge is also recognised (Margetson, 1997).

These attributes, while making PBL a desirable option, may also pose a threat for teachers comfortable with the traditional subject-based curricula. In PBL, teachers become facilitators of learning. It is the student's responsibility to learn. Lecturers must also change their role and 'let go', allowing students to explore issues of interest to them. A shift towards student-centred learning may bring anxieties related to a loss of lecturer control.

These are often expressed as concerns over what the students will actually learn if they do not receive lectures and/or tutorials covering the entire syllabus, and may cause resentment towards PBL and those members of staff engaged in it.

No matter how 'hot' teaching activity is, there is no guarantee that students will actually learn from it. With the expansion of health-based knowledge, subject-based nursing and midwifery courses (in common with many others) became more overcrowded as teachers attempted to cover more and more ground. Courses with a subject base often lack flexibility and are quickly out of date; topics are frequently taught in isolation and the programme becomes fragmented. This 'coveritis' creates confusion in the students, who may not see the relevance of topics to other subjects or indeed to professional practice. Students are passive participants in the process, may feel overloaded and may resort to learning only what is necessary to pass assignments.

PBL, on the other hand, gives students control over their own learning, sets the learning in a context in which it will be used, thus improving recall, spreads the learning load, and recognises existing knowledge and experience and their application. PBL, in its several guises, attempts to link reflective professional practice with a humanistic methodology of education to develop highly competent practitioners who will continue to learn effectively throughout their lives (Boud and Feletti, 1997) (cf. Chapter 1).

Historical background

The modern history of PBL dates back to the mid-1960s with the setting up of a PBL course in medicine at McMaster University, Hamilton, Ontario. Neufeld and Barrows (1974) suggest that the method is, in fact, much older and is loosely based on the tutorial system at Oxford University, which dates back to medieval times. McMaster University is itself uncertain how the PBL system actually developed. It acknowledges the work carried out at Case Western University in the USA in the 1950s, where a variety of educational strategies, including case histories and a multidisciplinary laboratory, were introduced to the undergraduate medical programme. Neufeld *et al.* (1989) tell of the desire to move away from the compartmentalisation of knowledge and the constant battles for ownership of the course content. Problems identified with the 1950s medical programme included a lack of integration of knowledge; an overdependence on 'teaching' – particularly by lecture – and attempting to teach everything in an effort to keep up with the growth of specialisms. Added to this was the realisation that knowledge was rapidly superseded by progress and that the course structure made it difficult to be innovative and responsive to the changes. The problems identified are still familiar to those engaged in healthcare education 40 years later.

A philosophy evolved at McMaster that aimed to reduce lectures, present basic sciences together with clinical problems, provide the opportunity for students to ask questions and enter into discussion, and create a course that would have the flexibility to vary the presentation of problems in response to changes in healthcare needs. The objectives for the courses reflected the desire to produce graduates who would be able to direct their own learning and would possess critical thinking and analytical skills which would be used to provide effective, efficient, humane care.

PBL reached Europe in 1971, when the newly created Medical Faculty at the University of Limburg in Maastricht, The Netherlands began a problem-based undergraduate medical programme. From this, the Maastricht '7 Jump' format was developed, a series of stages that slightly extends Barrows' closed loop process. (Schmidt, 1983). Students are asked to:

1. Clarify terms and concepts not readily understood
2. Define the problem
3. Analyse the problem (brainstorm)
4. Discuss and organise ideas inferred from step 3
5. Generate learning issues
6. Collect information outside the tutorial group
7. Report on and synthesise the newly acquired information.

The technique is more structured than the process begun at McMaster and has been widely adopted in European and Scandinavian countries, notably in the joint healthcare preparation programmes at Linköping in Sweden.

Since the introduction of the first course in 1969, PBL courses have developed across the globe and have spread from medicine to a range of other professions, including law, engineering, architecture, the police and social work. PBL has also been introduced into secondary education. Other healthcare professions were quick to perceive the benefits of employing a problem-based approach to learning. The 1970s and 80s saw an almost evangelical PBL movement as many institutions adopted the method almost as a matter of faith (Boud and Feletti, 1997). From this came a wealth of published material, mainly anecdotal, extolling the virtues of PBL. The 1990s brought a shift towards more rigorous research into a method that, superficially at least, seemed to offer no better results than traditional teaching, but that appeared to have a wide charismatic appeal. Much of the PBL material published in the 1990s generally supports the anecdotal reports from the 1980s. There is very little anti-PBL literature. Vernon (1995) suggests that this may be because of a reluctance to advertise failure when the rest of world is apparently succeeding. The volume of pro-PBL material is so large, however, that is unlikely that a similar amount of material against the process is lying unpublished.

The World Health Organization (WHO) (1993) and the World Bank (1993) each recommend PBL as an educational strategy that has much to offer as it reflects the environment in which healthcare professionals will work and is responsive to service needs. It is seen as having three educational objectives: the acquisition of an integrated body of knowledge related to commonly occurring health problems; the development or application of problem-solving skills; and the learning of clinical reasoning skills, which are particularly valuable in training healthcare professionals for community work. The English National Board for Nursing, Midwifery and Health Visiting (ENB) (1998) concludes that E(P)BL assists in the promotion of evidence-based practice as students are aware that nursing interventions must be underpinned by scrutiny of the research-based evidence.

With time, as PBL has spread from McMaster University to other cultures and courses, PBL has developed many variants, leading to much debate and occasional confusion on what does and what does not constitute PBL. Albanese and Mitchell (1993, p. 53), in a review of the literature on the outcomes and implementation of PBL, found defining PBL to be 'a confusing and somewhat contentious task'. PBL is not static, continuing to change and evolve as it is applied to an increasing number of disciplines and situations. Vernon and Blake (1993), in a review of PBL courses, found that PBL is more than a simple teaching strategy. They describe it as:

> A complex mixture of a general teaching philosophy, learning objectives and goals and faculty attitudes and values all of which are difficult to regulate and are often not well defined in research reports. (p. 560)

Such a complex mixture makes an evaluation of the PBL process difficult. The characteristics of PBL that appear to be most highly valued by students and PBL facilitators, and that provide the best examples, are often multidimensional and diverse, making it extremely difficult to pinpoint exactly why PBL is so successful and well accepted. Factual measures such as student success in national examinations indicate that there is little difference between students following traditional courses and students following PBL courses (Albanese and Mitchell, 1993). It is not possible to ascribe any apparent degree of success by one group or the other to the teaching methodology as there must always be differences between educational institutions. Even where institutions offer both PBL and traditional pathways, the differences in straightforward outcome measures do not explain the popularity of PBL even in comparison with other small-group or problem-solving approaches.

Approaches to implementing PBL

The dissemination of the PBL philosophy from McMaster University brought a series of adaptations in its wake as other institutions altered the PBL process to meet the needs of their own courses, students, resources and community. Several of the adaptations moved away from the original 'pure' PBL concept towards guided discovery learning, directed learning or case-based learning. These methods do not possess the all essential PBL characteristics (small groups, the presentation of a contextualised problem *prior* to learning, students' identification of their own learning needs, student seeking of content and subsequent feedback to the group), although they may demonstrate one or more of these. Other strategies similar to PBL, for example IBL (Feletti, 1993) and TBL (Harden *et al.*, 1996), also evolved.

Approaches to implementing PBL run along several continua: 'pure' to 'hybrid' PBL; uniform to single-strand PBL; homogeneous to parallel-track PBL; and in-school to out-school PBL. The amount of facilitator involvement, the degree of subject expertise possessed by the facilitator, the type of material used as a trigger for learning and the resources available will also influence the implementation method. The selections made from each of the various groupings will obviously create a range of PBL 'models' that will differ from one other even though still retaining the overall characteristics of PBL.

Pure versus hybrid PBL

Pure PBL follows the guidelines developed by McMaster University and expanded by Barrows. It is widely used in medical education. Students work in groups of approximately five with a facilitator. The group is presented with a problem set in a context that students will be likely to encounter in practice. Following a discussion of student-identified issues, the individual group members seek information about these identified issues. At the next meeting, the information is fed back to the group, and further discussion then takes place in order to reach a solution to the original problem. There are no formal lectures or tutorials, although students may contact subject specialists for advice. Barrows (1986) states that the hypothetico-deductive process undertaken by the students promotes the development of sound clinical reasoning skills, essential to medical practice.

Camp (1996, p. 3) reports on an email discussion in which the characteristics of 'pure' PBL were devised, namely that, for the learner, 'problem-based learning is active, adult-orientated, problem-centred, student-centred, collaborative, integrated, interdisciplinary, utilises small groups and operates in a clinical context'. Speaking at Brunel University in 1997, Barrows added the descriptors inquiry-based, self-directed, reiterative, self-reflective, self-motivated and practice-based to the list.

This list of characteristics replaced an earlier definition which claimed that programmes in which students are not in tutorial groups of 5–10, or in which PBL operates only in one part of the programme, cannot be regarded as 'pure' PBL. Many supporters of PBL who run programmes which do not meet all of the 'pure' characteristics – so-called 'hybrid' forms of PBL – also have much to offer. In hybrid models of PBL, 'fixed resource' sessions are added to assist in learning. The number and content of such sessions varies greatly. Some hybrid models include set laboratory and clinical skills sessions. Lectures and/or tutorials may be offered on topics considered to be essential or difficult to grasp. In some institutions, the lectures/tutorials are run at student request on topics decided by them. Question and answer sessions with subject experts may also be planned. One risk of hybrid PBL models is that institutions may adopt a 'belt and braces' approach in which the major issues that the PBL session is designed to trigger are also covered in lecture or tutorial sessions. Students quickly realise that little self-directed study is needed as lecturers will provide the answers. It is thus the PBL sessions that are perceived to be irrelevant to the factual leaning required by other sessions, and the deep learning benefits of PBL are lost. Sadlo (1997) found that occupational therapy students on hybrid PBL courses rated their course experience not only lower than that of those on 'pure' PBL courses, but also lower than that of students on subject-based courses for clarity of objectives and student inter-action. Findings by Kaufman and Mann (1996) indicate that student interaction may be less on PBL courses as the PBL groups tend to form cliques.

Uniform versus single-strand PBL

PBL may be implemented uniformly throughout a course or indeed may be used in every programme offered by an educa-tion institution (whole-school PBL); alternatively, it may be employed in only one module, one year, by one department or in relation to one topic area. Uniform implementation offers certain advantages: students are accustomed to PBL lessening the dissonance that may be experienced when moving from traditional learning to PBL (Moore-West *et al.*, 1989). There are also cost-benefits associated with resourcing across the institution. Evidence submitted to the ENB in 1998 indicated that the benefits of PBL were increased when it was implemented across a whole course.

Many centres begin the implementation of PBL in one module or in one department. Where this is part of an incremental process whereby the whole course moves towards uniform PBL, there are benefits related to an increased amount of time available for facilitator training, and to ensuring that the necessary support materials are *in situ*. Incremental implementation also allows start-up costs to be spread over 2 or more years. While partial implementation can have similar benefits in that fewer facilitators and resources are required, there are, however, pitfalls associated with limiting PBL to part of a course. Without the necessary support from the top, the module may be set up to fail. Facilitators need to be *au fait* with the PBL process, and sufficient suitable accommodation is needed for the PBL groups. Reyers (1997) tells of the difficulty of running a PBL module within a veterinary medicine course in a building where the only teaching accommodation was either a lecture theatre with seating for 120 students or a practical laboratory. Not surprisingly, many of the PBL sessions ended up being run in the cafeteria.

Where PBL is offered only in single module or by only one department, that topic may be perceived by students as being a soft option or of lesser value than traditionally taught subjects, particularly when the assessment is radically different. Students may also have problems in adapting to the self-directed learning style of PBL if they are accustomed to a knowledge-giving, lecture-based mode of teaching. This may create anxieties related to finding material and being sure that they are learning the 'right' thing.

Another format of 'single-strand' PBL is the use of problem-based sessions as integrators. PBL is used to apply topics learned by traditional methods to the context in which the student will need to use them. Although several institutions report employing PBL in this way, insufficient detail is available to decide whether or not the technique is in fact PBL or a problem-solving or case-study approach (Vernon and Blake, 1993).

Homogeneous or parallel track PBL

Homogeneous PBL courses are those in which all the students on the programme participate in PBL. This non-selective entry is typical of many PBL healthcare courses. When all students take part in the PBL process, there is a heavy demand on facilitators and resources – a difficulty that is particularly applicable to preregistration nursing programmes following the transfer of nurse education into the higher education sector.

An examination of differing individual adult learning styles, such as those identified by Entwhistle and Ramsden (1983) and Honey and Mumford (1992), suggests that PBL may not be a suitable learning method for all students, particularly where the course tends towards the 'purer' form of PBL. A proportion of students may dislike the team-work involved and prefer to learn solely through their own efforts. Others may find that practical 'hands-on' experience provides the favoured climate for learning match. Institutions that offer PBL courses may have different entry criteria and seek specific attributes to the standard academic entry requirements. In an attempt to meet the different student learning styles, while reducing the resourcing required for PBL, several institutions, usually medical schools, run 'parallel-track' PBL. In this situation, both PBL courses and traditionally taught courses leading to the same qualification are offered. Students state which type of course they would prefer at the time of application. The final selection for entry to the PBL courses is made by the faculty. Students not accepted for the PBL track enter the 'traditional' pathway. Although not explicitly stated, the need for faculty selection over and above self-selection suggests that the PBL pathways are oversubscribed.

Whatever the curriculum design used to implement PBL, support from the top management level in the organisation is essential for its success (Little and Sauer, 1997). Although the PBL philosophy is based on the individual learning needs of students, and allows the freedom for each student to explore his or her own areas of interest linked to the scenarios, the institutional structure required to resource PBL seems to need to be fairly rigid and inflexible. Institutions that have a long experience in running PBL courses, such as the University of Limburg and McMaster University, operate on well-defined matrix management structures.

In-school versus out-school PBL

PBL is used most often in the theoretical part of a programme, albeit within a practical context. Where the profession, be it engineering or nursing, requires the student to learn essential psychomotor skills in addition to cognitive skills, these are often taught in laboratories or clinical skills centres before the student is exposed to the 'live' situation. The need to acquire these skills is triggered by the use of PBL. Additionally, students are expected to identify when skills already learned would be applicable in different contexts in subsequent PBL scenarios.

Harden *et al.* (1996) advocate TBL as a strategy for teaching undergraduate medical students. TBL is similar to PBL in that small groups of students are presented with a problem and are required, through discussion, to identify issues and learning needs, undertake self-directed learning and then feed back to the group, but TBL has its own additional, unique attributes. In TBL, an essential task, for example patient assessment, is used as the trigger. The task is used to provide focus and context, but learning the task itself is not one of the learning outcomes of the TBL. Instead, the students explore the contexts in which the skill may be used. These increase in complexity as the students progress through the course and the skill is applied to a range of settings. Therefore, in their second year, students may learn about taking a history from a patient with chest pain. In subsequent years, this develops into the management of patients with, for example, acute myocardial infarction. Harden *et al.* (1996) state that TBL is a method promoting the acquisition of knowledge for its own sake and encouraging the development of higher learning objectives, rather than simply test-passing recall. This approach combines in-school theoretical learning with the clinical skills required for out-school practice.

The Hogeschool Limburg at Sittard in The Netherlands utilises PBL in an 'out-school' format. PBL, in the familiar format of the presentation of preprepared contextualised problems, is used during the students' theory time. During clinical practice periods, students come into school for sessions of reflection. As part of the reflective process, students are asked to identify a problem situation. After discussion, one of the problems from practice is selected as the PBL trigger for the PBL team (Heijnen, 1997).

It can be argued that this method resembles work-based learning rather than PBL. Triggers that appear to work best for student learning are those which 'smell real'. Problems that arise from the students' practical experience will certainly 'smell real'. This use of PBL in placements will be familiar to many nursing or midwifery lecturers who have, or have had, a clinical teaching remit. The selection of a patient-centred issue forms the basis for identifying the students' knowledge base and assists them in identifying their learning needs. The comfortable fit with clinical teaching techniques is one attribute that makes PBL an attractive method in the education of nursing students.

PBL facilitators

Teachers in PBL are often referred to as either 'tutors' or 'facilitators' as the role is one of guiding and assisting students, rather than of providing all the answers. The degree to which the facilitator interacts with the PBL group and the subject expertise of the facilitator are also variables in the PBL model. Facilitators may be present through each and every PBL session, or they may be present only for the feedback session. The interventions used by facilitators also vary. Some facilitators adhere closely to the tutorial skills of modelling higher-order thinking through asking questions that probe students' knowledge deeply and challenge learners' thinking, asking them to justify their assertions (Barrows, 1986), while others interact very little, intervening only when there is disjunction (cf. Chapter 6). The facilitator may remain with the PBL group throughout the programme, often acting as personal or academic tutor for the students within the group. The composition of the group remains relatively constant apart from losses resulting from attrition.

The facilitator is not a specialist in every topic identified in the PBL scenarios but does possess well-developed facilitation skills. Margetson (1997) states that PBL facilitation is simply good teaching and does not require skills specific to PBL. There is some debate over this, witnessed by the number of institutions that offer PBL facilitator training courses. Other PBL adherents recommend that each PBL session should be led by a subject specialist. Students are thus exposed to a variety of facilitators through their course and become accustomed to facilitators who 'know all the answers'. The latter method has the advantage of limiting personality clashes between facilitator and student.

The composition of the PBL group may also change with every new subject. While this has the advantage of limiting potential dysfunction in groups, it means that time is spent on group-building with every change of topic. Where the groups are changed, the question arises of who decides on the new group composition. Students are initially allocated to groups on a wholly or partially random basis, as few institutions know their new entrants well enough to gauge which students will work best together. Where there is a change of grouping, should students be allowed to make their own choices? Student selection fits with the PBL philosophy of student-centred learning, but there are risks in leaving the decision solely to students. While students who work well together will form well-functioning groups, there is a risk that students not selected by classmates will end up in a group that has a great potential for dysfunction.

The issue of group size is raised by Feletti (1993). He states that the pure form of hypothetico-deductive PBL advocated by Barrows (1986) and widely used in medical education is not particularly suited to nurse education. The suggested group number for this approach is given as four or five, although later papers by Barrows (1988, 1997) increase the number to eight. Given that the number of nurses being prepared for practice is considerably larger than the number of medical students, this small group size is unlikely to be feasible. Principles related to small-group work in general indicate that groups of between seven and 12 tend to perform optimally across a range of group tasks such as problem-solving, participation, cohesion and individual productivity (Curzon, 1985). McMaster University claims that it is possible to operate in PBL mode with groups of up to 150 students provided that students face each other with the teacher in the centre. Few institutions, however, currently possess McMaster University's wealth of experience.

Nursing students are also perceived to be less academically able than medical students. These differences, Feletti (1993) states, make E/IBL a better option for nurse education. E/IBL offers more flexibility of methods and a wider range of activities that can be triggered. It places less emphasis on teaching specific 'diagnostic' strategies, adopting a broader approach that allows for the consideration of 'messy' problems, which, Feletti claims, are more likely to be encountered by nurses. E/IBL places a greater emphasis on reflection and critical appraisal of the learning process than on access, analysing and synthesising material. It is possible to run E/IBL with groups of 20 or more, with a reduced demand on resources. Where there is a shortage of facilitators, there are other facilitation designs that conserve the smaller group size, such as one teacher facilitating students in two or more smaller groups rather than facilitating one larger group, or increasing the amount of self-directed work for groups of students in later years. The ENB review of evidence-based and problem-based courses undertaken in 1998 indicated that schools of nursing frequently utilised the term 'evidence-based learning' as there was often a resistance to the term 'problem-based learning'. The rationale for the change in terminology was given as one of political correctness rather than a feeling that the PBL process was not suitable for nursing students.

Trigger material

The range of material used to 'trigger' student identification of learning needs is wide and varied. Many of the triggers are 'paper cases', which themselves come in a variety of forms ranging from a few lines outlining the scenario through patient notes to situation improvement packages, which provide students with an ongoing unfolding of a patient history, with its attendant issues. Video clips also make popular triggers. Games, story boards, cartoons, role-play, poetry, quotations from literature, items of equipment, pictures and photographs, audiotapes, music – the list is bounded only by the innovation of the teams who create the triggers.

Simulated patients as triggers are particularly appreciated by students. They have the benefit of 'feeling real' and can provide instant feedback to students, not only in response to questions, but also on aspects of students' performance such as attitude, non-verbal communication, phasing of questions and manual handling skills. Creating a bank of simulated patients has ethical and resource implications. The range of exposure to students, and the situations required of simulated patients, needs careful consideration. Preparation for the role and consent are essential. Even when simulated patients are unpaid volunteers, the costs related to preparing patients for their various roles and in maintaining records can be considerable.

Originality is not all, however. Trigger materials need rigorous evaluation to ensure that they do, in fact, stimulate the desired learning and do not send students off on tangents that, although interesting, do not relate to the course outcomes.

The possible permutations and combinations of design variables in PBL are endless. (Barrows, 1986, p. 483)

Pros and cons of PBL

While PBL offers several advantages for nurse/midwife education, there are also some drawbacks that require consideration both prior to and during implementation.

The structuring of knowledge for use in clinical contexts, the developing of an effective clinical reasoning process; the development of effective self-directed learning skills, and increased motivation for learning are proffered in support of the use of PBL. The increase in application of PBL and its transmission to disciplines other than medicine have led to additional claims being made about its benefits. PBL is claimed to enhance the acquisition, retention and use of knowledge, in addition to increasing its retrievability.

The basis for many of these claims lies in the ability of PBL to provide the conditions required to promote deep learning in students. The purpose of higher education (nursing and midwifery now being taught within the higher education structure) is to promote higher levels of cognitive thinking (Margetson, 1994). Work by Entwhistle and Ramsden in the late 1970s and early 80s highlighted differences between surface approaches to learning and deep approaches to learning. The surface approach to learning is characterised by students memorising facts for assessment purposes, viewing learning as being imposed from the outside, failing to take responsibility for their own learning, focusing on individual topic areas without making links between subjects, and being motivated by external rewards (assignment results). Factors that promote a surface learning approach are linked to the traditional subject-based curriculum, which tends towards teacher direction with too many passive learning situations, for example lectures, too many assessments that test only quantity of knowledge rather than quality of thought, and an overloaded curriculum as teachers strive to 'cover' all there is to know. Students feel that studying becomes an imposition and an irrelevance in their lives.

Where deep approaches to learning are adopted, the student attempts to understand the subject, tries to relate new learning to existing knowledge and previous experience, examines the argument, and is motivated to learn for its own sake. Biggs (1988) identified four conditions that foster a deep approach to learning – motivational context, learner activity, interaction with others and a well-structured knowledge base. PBL has the potential to fulfil all of these criteria (Patel *et al.*, 1991).

Over the years, PBL has been credited with many positive attributes that are particularly attractive to the education of healthcare workers (WHO, 1993). In addition to the creation of clinical reasoning and self-directed learning skills, PBL is also credited with improving presentation and feedback skills, promoting team-working and, through discussion and argument in group settings, encouraging students to justify their decisions (Albanese and Mitchell, 1993).

At the end of the twentieth century, much debate arose in the UK over whether nursing should return to an 'on-the-job' style of 'training' and abandon the academic pathway. If this were to occur, there would be little opportunity for an in-depth study of topics, which would result in the loss of adaptability in the workforce, something that the government views as an outcome of a higher education.

PBL is neither uniformly superior nor invariably successful, an argument often raised by antagonists of PBL. Research indicates that students from PBL-style courses do not perform any better in national examinations, such as licensing examinations, than students from traditionally taught courses, particularly in basic science subjects (Albanese and Mitchell, 1993; Vernon and Blake, 1993). Initial recall is poorer than that seen in students taught by more traditional methods, although this finding is misleading as it is difficult to test what has been learned when PBL students identify their own learning. Given that PBL does not promote the memorisation of factual material for test-passing, it is perhaps more surprising that the performance of PBL students is no worse than that of traditionally taught students.

It has been questioned whether PBL is worth the effort and cost related to the extra teaching and other resources involved. Research (Martensen *et al.*, 1985; Norman and Schmidt, 1992) indicates that learning through PBL lasts longer than learning by traditional methods and that learning is likely to continue after qualification. Shin *et al.* (1993) found that PBL course doctors had more up-to-date knowledge in the years after graduation compared with graduates from traditionally taught medical courses. Doctors from PBL courses showed no correlation between the length of time from graduation and the currency of their knowledge, whereas colleagues from traditional courses demonstrated a negative correlation between the time since graduation and up-to-date knowledge. Shin *et al.* suggest that the self-directed learning skills fostered by PBL helped to offset the effects of ageing on memory. Given that students currently on nursing courses will, hopefully, still be working in the 2030s, and that nursing knowledge will have expanded and developed in that time, lifelong learning skills are vital. PBL offers a method of meeting the need to develop lifelong learning skills advocated in the Dearing and Garrick reports on higher education (1997).

The relevance of material is also important, the 'smells real' factor being one of the major strengths of PBL. The ability of PBL to set material in a context in which it will be used in practice offers several benefits. The curriculum becomes more flexible and meaningful to the students, and epidemiological shifts and advances in treatments can be easily incorporated. The contextualisation allows for the integration of several topics into a situation that is pertinent to the student. Dissonance between the present curriculum and the student's future role is reduced. In addition, the development of self-motivated learning overcomes feelings of overload and too much to be learned in too short a time. Although the evidence suggests that PBL students do not perform well in basic sciences, there is some indication that the integration of basic sciences with clinical sciences is, in fact, improved. Albanese and Mitchell (1993) report that the clinical performance of PBL students is well rated, particularly in areas where sound team-working and well developed communication skills are particularly required.

In addition to the benefits that PBL produces for future practice, much of the material on PBL emphasises its advantages with respect to the actual student experience. PBL is reported as being positively rated by students, especially where students have self-selected to undertake a PBL course. The use of small groups, the emphasis on the self-identification of learning needs, and the opportunity to discuss issues contribute to increased student interest, personal satisfaction, increased attendance at classes and enhanced interpersonal skills. Student–staff communication and relationships are improved by the close contact of a small group of students with one staff member. This aspect has particular attraction for Adult branch teachers as it offers the opportunity to know a small group of students well. PBL is credited with an improvement in student reasoning, but the influences of different faculties make this aspect difficult to assess (Vernon and Blake, 1993; Sadlo 1997).

The enjoyment generated by PBL for both students and tutors is perhaps the most striking attribute to emerge from the literature. Irrefutable evidence fully to support PBL as the superior teaching strategy has yet to emerge, but there is little doubt that it is a most enjoyable experience and, as a result, generates interest and enthusiasm. Norman and Schmidt (1992) found that PBL tends to be run by teachers who enjoy PBL and that the process is therefore self-generating. Teachers who obviously enjoy teaching tend to be highly rated by students, regardless of course design.

Kaufman and Mann (1996), in a study comparing medical students on a PBL course with those on the traditional medical programme, found that the PBL course students had increased enthusiasm for the curriculum, finding it stimulating and enjoyable, exciting curiosity and providing information essential to their future role. Evidence to the ENB (1998) reported that preregistration students on PBL/EBL courses reported increased confidence in dealing with complex issues. Reflection in practice becomes second nature as students develop the ability to think through practice issues in a reasoned way. The focus within PBL on independent and interdependent working reflects practice.

Despite the volume of literature in favour of PBL, there are certain drawbacks that must be taken into consideration when planning a PBL curriculum. It has been suggested that the reported successes of PBL may be due to a form of the Hawthorne effect or to teacher-pleasing strategies that lead students to report positively on PBL. Problem-based courses may attract different types of students, ones who would develop critical thinking and lifelong learning skills regardless of which type of course they followed (Vernon and Blake, 1993).

There may be a feeling that existing breadth in a programme has been sacrificed to permit students to undertake in-depth study. PBL proponents argue that students should be presented with the situations they are most likely to encounter in practice, and that through discussion of issues related to these, they will develop the techniques needed to manage the more rarely occurring situations; for example, nursing students in the UK may be presented with a scenario related to the nursing care required by a patient with a suprapubic catheter. An exploration of this scenario, and an identification and justification of the nursing actions required, will assist them in deciding the nursing interventions required for a patient with a Mitrofanoff valve.

This raises the question of the student's ability to transfer knowledge learned in one situation to another. Work undertaken by Needham and Begg (1991) indicates that feedback is the key factor. The discussion that takes place during PBL feedback sessions should enable students to develop transferable skills if sound feedback is received. If developing higher levels of cognitive thinking is the educationalist's aim of higher education, the development of transferable skills for a flexible workforce is the aim of the government. PBL has the potential to develop both.

The demand on staff members where there is a large number of students is heavy, whether the load is spread over a large number of staff or focused on a smaller number who facilitate a larger number of student teams. If the latter, fewer teachers are available for other teaching requirements. In addition to teacher resources, there is also a requirement for additional supporting material, particularly access to library resources, including computerised databases and the Internet. Other resources may include access to subject experts both within the institution and in related practice areas. Additionally, disciplines that have a skills aspect to their practice will need to provide suitable environments where skills can be practised safely. For nurse and midwife education, this has implications for the provision of clinical skills laboratories. Students on courses employing PBL may require open access to clinical skills laboratories outside teacher-arranged sessions. At a purely logistical level, sufficient rooms in which to run PBL sessions are required. There are also time constraints. It will take longer for students to find things out for themselves than for someone to do the searching for them and convey the information in lecture format. However, Boud and Feletti (1997) indicate that no link has been shown between the degree of resourcing and the success of PBL.

PBL does not suit every student. As learning styles are individual, the emphasis on finding, sharing and discussing material may not fit everyone and may lead to some student discomfort (Vermunt and van Rijswijk, 1988). This applies equally to other teaching strategies and may be partially offset in PBL by the use of other methods, such as lectures, laboratory work and open learning materials in fixed resource sessions. Students on PBL courses require to shift their view of teachers. Traditional school education tends to present teachers as disseminators of knowledge, students being passive recipients who have 'lost the ability to wonder'. In PBL, the responsibility for learning is placed firmly with the student – the regurgitation of lecture notes being insufficient. Moore-West *et al.* (1989) report that although students always experienced some distress and dissonance during a medical programme, this was always less for PBL students. Recent work with medical and nursing students (Dolmans and Schmidt, 1994; Jacobsen, 1997) indicates that students develop their own agendas and that these 'frame factors' – which may or may not be related to the course work – can interfere with the intended learning regardless of the quality of facilitation.

Assessment is a major issue in PBL (cf. Chapter 7). Many of the traditional assignments, for example examinations, do not fit well with PBL as they rely on memory rather than critical thinking. Developing expertise in assignments such as the Triple Jump exercise takes time and effort.

Although firmly set in practice contexts, PBL is a cognitive strategy: nursing is a practice-based vocation; learning that takes place in practice is more powerful.

The popularity of PBL has also come under attack. It is not important for students to like their work: enjoyment does not equal quality. It would seem, however, that this maxim is not always applied equitably across institutions, but is instead singled out for application to PBL. Conversely, a lack of enjoyment does not equal quality.

Conclusion

PBL is a technique that offers nursing/midwifery students the opportunity to adopt a deep learning approach to identifying problematic issues, recognising their individual learning needs, organising themselves to acquire relevant knowledge and applying it to the situation (cf. Chapter 9). The strategy allows lecturers of nursing and midwifery to construct courses reflecting current health needs in a context in which they will be encountered by students in practice. The process is resource intensive, and it will not suit the learning styles of all students. Success requires continued managerial support, meticulous advance planning and preparation, and a continuous supply of motivated facilitators. If this is not maintained, there is a danger that PBL will become routine and thus poorly implemented. More empirically based research is needed to identify (to paraphrase Graham Feletti) 'What works and what doesn't in PBL in nurse/midwife education.'

Implementing PBL takes hard work and commitment at all levels – it cannot be regarded as a 'quick fix' (Margetson, 1997). The work, although hard, is enjoyable. PBL has the potential to respond rapidly to changes in professional knowledge and to promote evidence-based practice and team-working, all valuable attributes for a career as a qualified nurse or midwife.

PBL glossary

Facilitator: a member of teaching staff allocated to a PBL team to assist in working through the situation and to help with identifying learning needs. The facilitator will neither provide answers nor give tutorials to the team, but will assist them in focusing on their learning requirements. As the programme progresses, students will be encouraged to become proficient and independent in identifying learning needs associated with situations and in transferring these techniques to practice.

Facilitator package: a set of identical material provided for each facilitator by the lecturers who compile the situation. This should contain student and lecturer objectives, references, expected questions/answers, facilitator and student evaluation/reflection forms and so on.

Fixed resource: additional material available to the student to assist with learning. Fixed resources take a variety of forms, for example lectures, tutorials, clinical skills sessions, open learning packages, computer assisted learning programmes, journal articles, books, videos and so on.

Learning activity: an exercise designed to promote learning through, for example, discussion, searching/reviewing material or practical experimentation.

PBL session: the time when the PBL team meet to decide on the learning needs associated with the given situation. The work required to fulfil the identified needs is allocated to team members through negotiation. Sessions may be introductory when the situation is first presented; intermediate where learning is reviewed and learning needs to be reassessed; or feedback sessions in which each member of the team presents his or her contribution towards the team's learning. Sessions may or may not be facilitated.

PBL team: students who meet together, on a regular basis throughout the programme, with the purpose of learning about a series of situations that mirror practice.

Portfolio: the student's personal file, which contains a record of the learning achieved from each situation.

Problem: the situation may be presented as a problem that has to be worked through.

Problem-based learning (PBL): an educational strategy using material that is as close as possible to real life as a stimulus for learning. It takes account of *how* people learn. Learners are actively engaged and involved with the material. Learning to develop lifelong enquiry and learning skills is more important than remembering content.

Problem-solving approach: an approach to the delivery of individualised midwifery/nursing care that the student will encounter during clinical experience.

Resource box: a box available to each team for each situation. This will contain items such as research articles, manufacturers' information, literature, videos and small items of equipment.

Scenario: the detail related to the situation. This may or may not form part of the trigger.

Situation: reflects a true-to-life practice experience that requires certain knowledge and skills in order to provide nursing/midwifery care for the patient/client. Students identify what relevant knowledge they have already and determine what they need to learn in relation to the given situation.

Situation improvement package (SIP): a collection of additional material relating to the patient/client in the scenario. The material may be introduced incrementally.

Trigger: the initial stimulus used to introduce each situation. These will vary greatly in nature, being for example, nursing/midwifery notes, video clips and so on.

References

Albanese, M A and Mitchell, S (1993) Problem-based Learning: A Review of Literature on its Outcomes and Implementation Issues, *Academic Medicine,* **68**(1): 52–81.

Barrows, H S (1986) A Taxonomy of Problem-based Learning Methods, *Medical Education,* **20**: 481–6.

Barrows, H S (1988) *The Tutorial Process,* Springfield, IL: Southern Illinois University School of Medicine.

Barrows, H S (1997) Challenges of Changing from Subject-based to Problem-based Learning, Paper Changing to PBL, International Conference on Problem-based Learning, Brunel University, September.

Barrows, H S and Tamblyn, R M (1980) *Problem-based Learning: An Approach to Medical Education,* New York: Springer.

Biggs, J B (1988) The Role of Metacognition in Enhancing Learning, *Australian Journal of Education,* **32**(2): 127–38.

Biley, F (1998) Evaluating a Welsh Nursing Education PBL Programme: A Short Report, *Probe,* **18**: 12–13.

Boud, D and Feletti, G I (eds) (1997) *The Challenge of Problem-based Learning* (2nd edn), London: Kogan Page.

Camp, G (1996) Problem-based Learning: A Paradigm Shift or Passing Fad? *Medical Education Outline,* **1**: 2.

Curzon, L B (1985) *Teaching in Further Education: An Outline of Principles and Practice* (3rd edn), London: Cassell Educational.

Dolmans, D H J M and Schmidt, H G (1994) What Drives the Student in Problem-based Learning? *Medical Education,* **28**: 372–80.

English National Board for Nursing, Midwifery and Health Visiting (1998) D*evelopments in the Use of an Evidence and/or Enquiry Based Approach in Nursing, Midwifery and Health Visiting Programmes of Education,* http://www.enb.org.uk/evidpub.htm.

Entwhistle, N J and Ramsden, P (1983) *Understanding Student Learning,* London: Croom Helm.

Feletti, G I (1993) Inquiry Based and Problem Based Learning: How Similar are these Approaches to Nursing and Medical Education?, *Higher Education Research and Development,* **12**(2): 143–56.

Harden, R M, Laidlaw, J M, Kerr, J S and Mitchell, H E (1996) Task-based Learning: An Educational Strategy for Undergraduate, Postgraduate and Continuing Medical Education, Parts 1 & 2, *Medical Teacher,* **18**(1): 7–13; **18**(2): 91–8.

Heijnen, R (1997) The In-school and Out-school Learning Process According to PBL, Paper Changing to PBL, International Conference on Problem-based Learning, Brunel University, September.

Honey, P and Mumford, A (1992) *The Manual of Learning Styles* (3rd edn), Maidenhead: Peter Honey.

Jacobsen, D Y (1997) Tutorial process in a problem-based learning context; medical students' reception and negotiations. Unpublished thesis, Norwegian University of Science and Technology.

Kaufman, D M and Mann, K V (1996) Comparing Students' Attitudes in Problem-based and Conventional Curricula, *Academic Medicine*, **71**: 1096–9.

Little, S E and Sauer, C (1997) Organizational and Institutional Impediments to a Problem-based Approach. In Boud, D and Feletti, G I (eds) (1997) *The Challenge of Problem-based Learning* (2nd edn), London: Kogan Page.

Margetson, D (1994) Current Educational Reform and the Significance of Problem-based Learning, *Studies in Higher Education*, **19**(1): 5–19.

Margetson, D (1997) Why is Problem-based Learning a Challenge? In Boud, D and Feletti, G I (eds) *The Challenge of Problem-based Learning*, (2nd edn), London: Kogan Page.

Martensen, D, Eriksson, H and Ingelman-Sundberg, M (1985) Medical Chemistry: Evaluation of Active and Problem-oriented Teaching Methods, *Medical Education*, **19**: 34–42.

Moore-West, M, Harrington, D L, Mennin, S P, Kaufman, A and Skipper, B J (1989) Distress and Attitudes towards the Learning Environment: Effects of a Curriculum Innovation, *Teaching and Learning in Medicine*, **1**(3): 151–7.

National Committee of Enquiry into Higher Education, (Chairman R Dearing) (1997a) *Higher Education in the Learning Society*, London: NCIHE.

National Committee of Enquiry into Higher Education, (Chairman R Garrick, Scottish Committee) (1997b) *Higher Education in the Learning Society: Report of the Scottish Committee*, Edinburgh: NCIHE.

Needham, D R and Begg, I M (1991) Problem-oriented Training Promotes Spontaneous Analogical Transfer. Memory Oriented Training Promotes Memory for Training, *Memory and Cognition*, **19**: 543–57.

Neufeld, V R and Barrows, H S (1974) The 'McMaster Philosophy': An Approach to Medical Education, *Journal of Medical Education*, **49**: 1040–50.

Neufeld, V R, Woodward, C A and MacLeod, S M (1989) The McMaster MD Program: A Case Study Renewal in Medical Education, *Academic Medicine*, **64**: 423–43.

Norman, G R and Schmidt, H G (1992) The Psychological Basis of Problem-based Learning: A Review of the Evidence, *Academic Medicine*, **67**: 557–65.

Patel, V L, Groen, G L and Norman, G R (1991) Effects of Conventional and Problem-based Medical Curricula on Problem-solving, *Academic Medicine*, **66**: 380–9.

Reyers, F (1997) PBL in a PBL-ignorant and PBL-hostile (logistically) Environment. Paper, International Conference on Problem-based Learning, Brunel University, September.

Sadlo, G (1997) Problem-based Learning Enhances the Educational Experiences of Occupational Therapy Students, *Education for Health*, **10**(1): 101–14.

Schmidt, H G (1983) Problem-based Learning: Rationale and Description, *Medical Education*, **17**: 11–16.

Shin, J H, Haynes, B, Johnston, M E (1993) Effect of Problem-based, Self-directed Undergraduate Education on Life Long Learning, *Canadian Medical Association Journal*, **148**(6): 969–76.

Vermunt, J D H M and Van Rijswijk, F (1988) Analysis and Development of Students' Skill in Self-regulating Learning, *Higher Education*, **17**: 647–82.

Vernon, D T A (1995) Attitudes and Opinions of Faculty Tutors about Problem-based Learning, *Academic Medicine*, **70**(3): 216–23.

Vernon, D T A and Blake, R L (1993) Does Problem-based Learning Work? A Meta-analysis of Educative Research, *Academic Medicine* **68**(7): 550–63.

World Bank (1993) *World Development Report 1993: Investing in Health*, Oxford: Oxford University Press.

World Health Organization (1993) *Increasing the Relevance of Education for Health Professionals*, Report of a WHO Study Group on Problem-solving Education for the Health Professionals, Technical Report Series No. 838, Geneva: WHO.

3

Preparation for Implementing Problem-based Learning

Carolyn Gibbon

Introduction

PBL was introduced into the School of Health at Liverpool John Moores University in June 1997 as a result of three events coming together. The first was the impending revalidation of preregistration nursing programmes. It was clear that there was a need to be innovative to link theory and practice more succinctly, and to manage large groups in a more coherent fashion. The second 'event' was the need to increase student activity in a practice-based discipline. The third event was the author attending a conference on PBL at McMaster University. PBL may be regarded as a philosophy or as a teaching and learning methodology (Alavi, 1995), and as such would fulfil these stated requirements (cf. Chapter 2). Time was limited, so the decision was taken to implement PBL into the integrated theory/practice modules that account for over half of the academic credits towards a diploma/degree in nursing. An enormous amount of preparation in terms of staff development, learning packs and assessment and evaluation strategies also took place. This chapter discusses how this School of Health introduced PBL into its preregistration nursing curriculum.

Staff development

The development of staff is a vital issue with any new innovation, and in relation to PBL, the literature supports this view (McMillan and Dwyer, 1989). The strategy for staff development evolved over time and followed initial contacts with colleagues in other universities. In order to give feedback to colleagues from the Canadian conference, two lunchtime seminars were held. The purpose of these was to provide feedback, to present staff with the idea of PBL and also to discuss how this methodology could be implemented. As anticipated, there was some scepticism, but there was also a great deal of enthusiasm. It was also noted that implementing an innovation such as this would require more than one person. Fortunately, a colleague was willing to assist.

Talking to colleagues and visiting other university sites proved beneficial. We were also 'visited', which boosted morale in that it demonstrated that we were not toying with the idea, but that this was a serious venture. Visitors questioning our development forced us to be reflective and hence strengthened our position. An interesting opportunity presented itself when a small group of people from across the wider university visited Manchester Medical School on a 'learning raid'. Other subject areas from the university were also demonstrating an interest in PBL, and our hosts on this occasion were generous in answering questions, allowing us the opportunity to sit in with groups in action, and in their hospitality. As our programme unfolds and more groups are using PBL, we are able to offer similar experiences to other colleagues external (as well as internal) to our school. The notion of 'swap-shop' is important for helping to form and consolidate ideas on how PBL may be introduced and implemented.

The information gleaned in this way was important to us in helping to formalise our ideas about how this process was implemented in the new curriculum. These thoughts culminated in a specific staff development strategy focusing on facilitation, informing and preparing clinical staff and developing learning materials. The strategy includes mechanisms for informal and formal feedback, as Doring *et al.* (1995) note that it is important for staff to feel comfortable with the process and their role. If this is absent, there will not be the support and co-operation that is needed for PBL to be implemented.

Facilitators

At present, all the facilitators are volunteers and it is the intention to continue with this situation for as long as possible. They are staff who have expressed a desire to be facilitators and have been involved in seminars and workshops. This raised resource issues (cf. Chapter 2). PBL can be lecturer intensive and strategies need to be employed to cope with this matter.

A series of hour-long seminars was organised, each discussing a different issue. These have now been largely superseded by interactive workshops lasting either a half-day or a whole day. The type of workshop depends on the topic in hand. The workshop for new facilitators is an all-day event. This gives participants the opportunity to work through a learning package and develop an overview of PBL. All participants are offered the chance to co-facilitate by working alongside an established facilitator. New facilitators are also given a copy of a Facilitator's Guide, which gives an overview of PBL and how the groups are formed. It also discusses how to run a group and how possibly to deal with students who may be disruptive. In light of our experiences over the past 12 months, the Guide is in the process of being updated to take into account local changes such as staff reorganisation, room changes and so on. All workshops are evaluated for the following reasons:

- To advise what further learning is needed
- To provide feedback on how the workshop was received
- To inform the implementation strategy.

There is an hour-long meeting of the facilitators' support group each Friday, which usually takes place in our Teaching and Learning Centre. There is only one item on the agenda – that of issues related to facilitation. Minutes are taken as a record of the meeting and occasionally used to refer to. Attendance is voluntary, facilitators sometimes not being able to attend because of pressures of work. However, the meeting provides an opportunity to discuss:

- Matters arising from facilitation.
- Opportunities for neophyte facilitators to team up with established facilitators.
- Opportunities for peer review.

This is especially important in relation to subject quality review, which will have taken place in all university-based nursing programmes by the year 2000.

Many facilitators have also found it useful to keep reflective diaries, based on a model of reflection (John, 1994). Students are also encouraged to keep diaries, so facilitators feel that they can act as a role model. The diaries are personal but can form the basis of discussion at the support group meeting. When exploring how the concept of change theory had taken place in practice, a number of facilitators kindly gave permission for information from their diaries to be examined and some parts used as evidence to support the use of PBL. This was very much appreciated and demonstrated that the strategy being employed to introduce PBL was developing satisfactorily.

All staff are kept informed of developments through an internal newsletter 'PBL News'. This contains feedback from specific workshops, events that have taken place or are about to take place in relation to PBL within the school, and other progress reports. The newsletter is produced every couple of months, staff always being encouraged to feed back on the editorial or other points raised.

Clinical staff

The development of clinical staff is a huge undertaking as students are allocated to placements that cover seven diverse Trusts and a multitude of Directorates. The pressures on clinical staff are enormous, and it is vital that academic staff are aware of these constraints. It was decided that a 'drip-feed' approach was the most suitable method to use. Toward this end, an overview of PBL was given to the senior nurse management in all of the Trusts. This was then followed up by a series of 2-hour workshops for staff. Putting these workshops into action has largely been brought about by liaising with clinical development nurses, who canvassed staff and discussed with ward managers releasing these staff to attend the workshops.

Clinical staff are given a briefing about PBL and how students receive their information via the learning packs. Examples are circulated and staff encouraged to comment. The main concern from the point of view of clinical staff is their feeling that students are going to be more informed than themselves. They have been reassured that this is not the case, and that the *experience* that clinical staff have will be valued and much sought after by the students. Staff are advised how a differing questioning technique may be employed in order to encourage students to seek information for themselves. They are also encouraged to follow the student's line of reasoning so that the student and the qualified nurse can gain the most from the experience. An overview of PBL is now included in the ENB 997/8 (Learning and Teaching Preparation for Practitioners) course, and (it is hoped) clinical staff return to base and discuss this with their clinical colleagues. In this way, a cascade effect will be produced both upwards and outwards.

Students are also encouraged to take their learning pack with them to their placement. Each student's learning pack contains the scenario under study, brief resource guidelines and room to write their findings (see below for further details). Initial concerns were that the pack bore no relation to the placement, as is sometimes the case. However, all packs have to meet the learning outcomes for the module, and there are identified concepts that should be applicable wherever the student is placed. By taking their packs to their placement, students can share their learning with their assessor/mentor; in this way, a real partnership in learning develops. The partnership is further enhanced as the facilitators will also visit their students in practice. These visits currently amount to one per semester, but the purpose is to check progress and encourage the development of active learning. The learning pack provides an ideal vehicle for this process. The expertise of clinical staff is invaluable in the development of learning packs. In our experience, we have found staff more than willing to assist in the writing of packs. Thus, theory and practice are truly linked, and the clinical staff feel a greater sense of ownership in relation to educational materials.

Learning packs

Learning packs are used to enable students to be facilitated through PBL.

A learning pack group was set up very early on, and guidance was sought from the literature (Hengstberger-Sims and McMillan, 1993) and through packs purchased from McMaster University. All the packs are based on actual patients/clients, as advised by the literature, the point being that the individual on whom the pack is based must be plausible. This is only possible if there are actual personal data related to them, with a clear clinical record of events. This also prevents disputes over what has taken place. Any disputes that do occur are rechannelled into discussions looking at the wider implications of why certain care did or did not take place. In our experience, especially with having a well-known children's hospital around the corner, it is vital that the 'case' is ordinary. Confidentiality must be respected, and an unusual case may attract unwanted attention (hence the relevance of the children's hospital). Over time, a house style has developed for the presentation of these packs to students, Table 3.1 being meant as a guide only. The services of a member of the Learning Resources Unit have been invaluable for this process, and the development of a template has considerably speeded up the process of pack production.

Each pack comprises two parts: a student pack and a facilitator pack. The student pack contains information related to the scenario, associated concepts, the learning outcomes for the module and a list of resources to point students in the right direction, as illustrated. The facilitator pack is, in effect, a supplementary pack and includes all the relevant data associated with the named individual in the pack. The resource guide that is included in all the packs comes about through the co-operation of a member of Learning Services. The guide includes key words for using CD-ROM and paper resources. People who may be willing to be approached and questioned by students are also included, as are the names of lay organisations who are willing to help (especially if booklets may be available). While this appears to be a fairly comprehensive list, each section may include only one or two names to trigger off students and hopefully enable them to seek more widely.

Table 3.1 Content of learning packs

Cover	Module details and name of pack (for example, Mary Shaw)
Page 1	Placement details (room for student to make notes)
Page 2	Learning outcomes for the module
Page 3	Scenario
Page 4	Related concepts
Page 5	Issues raised
Page 6	Possible explanations
Page 7	Learning needs
Page 8	Resource file (including search terms and so on)
Page 9	Fixed resource sessions (for the student to arrange and note)
Page 10	Care issues
Page 11	Action plan
Page 12	Evaluation of pack through reflection

In terms of administration there are a number of issues that need to be taken into account:

- The PBL module leaders have a responsibility, with a colleague acting as a 'pack co-ordinator', to develop the packs.

- A validation group, made up of representatives from across the school, discusses and 'validates' each pack. This group is led by the assistant director for preregistration courses.
- The pack co-ordinator is responsible for proof-reading the packs, ordering them from the print room and delivering them to the module facilitators.
- Modules are one semester long in this university, so each PBL module requires at least three packs to cover the learning outcomes.

Assessment

The need to reflect the PBL process is vital in terms of assessment (cf. Chapter 7). Altering assessments has been more difficult to implement as it is hard to let go of tried and tested methods. However, following evaluations from the first PBL module, it was found to be easier to change the assessment. While students still have to write an assignment, the title and structure of the assignment is now more in keeping with the work that they will have done in their module. The processes of reflection and integrating current research and practice developments are now more overt.

It is also worth noting that, at one time, all assignments to be marked were the responsibility of the module leader. The current intake of 170 students, however, made this an impossible task, so the responsibility of marking has now been devolved down to facilitators, the final mark being forwarded to the module leader. The effect of this is twofold:

- The facilitator has a better understanding of the student's learning.
- The facilitator's marking load has shifted from looking at a multitude of scripts from one module to marking a few scripts from a number of modules, depending which ones they are involved with. This enables a higher degree of marking quality and a better opportunity for quality feedback to the student, as well as a greater overview of the whole programme.

Clinical skills are also assessed through the use of objectively structured clinical assessment. In our school, this method of assessment is in its infancy. In discussions with clinical colleagues, this method of assessment is viewed as a positive move for a number of reasons:

● Students feel more comfortable in the clinical situation. Having been tested on key skills, they are able to work with a degree of independence.
● Clinical staff are more accepting of students with these skills. This is not staff abdicating their role as teachers of skills, but working in an often fraught situation where there is too much to do and too few staff to do it.

Evaluation

The importance of evaluation was noted right from the outset (cf. Chapter 7). All workshops are evaluated, the information provided forming the basis for ongoing staff development. Learning packs and the process of PBL are evaluated by the students as well. This information also includes material about their facilitator that is returned to individual facilitators and is treated in a confidential manner. The facilitators evaluate the students' performance and the progress of the packs. Any short-comings are noted and reported back to the learning package validation group. Positive feedback is also welcomed. Needless to say, a huge amount of information has been generated and has been most useful for fine-tuning packs and so on. However, this information has needed to be streamlined, so an evaluation strategy was developed to prevent student and facilitator boredom. To illustrate this, imagine two groups A and B: group A students will evaluate packs 1 and 3, and in their next module, they will evaluate pack 2. Group B (who are in the next cohort) will evaluate pack 2, and then packs 1 and 3 in their next module.

The huge amount of data is in danger of being lost, and nego-tiations are currently underway to employ a research assistant, on a part-time basis, to catalogue this information. To some, this type of data collection may seem superficial, but we need to build on what information we have and compare notes with other institutions, a point that appears to be being actively encouraged by Biley (1998) in his report of an evaluation of a PBL nursing programme in Wales.

Pilot study

The opportunity arose whereby a colleague gave permission for her module to be used as a pilot study in PBL. This 6-month module was the final module of the 'old' diploma course, running alongside two other modules related to community nursing and nursing management. Students were divided into groups and introduced to PBL through a hypothetical patient – Mary Shaw – before moving on to actual situations. Each group was allocated by the lecturer, whereas subsequent groups have chosen themselves. This has raised some interesting situations in terms of group dynamics, but it was felt that there was a need to sort out the groups before moving on.

Students were assessed by the self-directed learning readiness scale (Gugliomeno, 1977) at the start and end of the module, these results currently being processed. During the module, as groups completed a pack, their individual contribution and how they rated the group-working were also evaluated. This was important as many students had never before been in the situation of peer review. All the packs were evaluated, as previously discussed, and the group process was also evaluated by the facilitator. Comparing the facilitators' evaluation with the groups' evaluation forms the basis for discussion and has made many students much more aware of their strengths and weaknesses. All PBL sessions ended with a brief feedback on performance, this being followed by a 'debriefing' session for facilitators. These meetings then developed into the facilitators' support group.

Altering the format of the module also entailed altering the assessment method. The pilot students undertook a three-part assessment:

- The group (approximately 15 students) was subdivided into three or four smaller groups. Each group gave a presentation that was peer marked, the facilitator acting as moderator.

- This presentation was then written up and formally marked by the facilitator.
- A final individual written assignment was submitted at the end of the module.

The pilot study was measured against criteria related to student learning outcomes, the depth and breadth of learning and also attendance. If judged in terms of assessment, the students were found to have performed better than previous cohorts undertaking a similar assignment (cf. Chapter 7). Depth and breadth were initially an issue as both facilitators and students were adjusting to the change in method. At the end of the pilot study, these had improved considerably, facilitators and students feeling much more satisfied with their outcomes, but clinical staff also provided anecdotal evidence stating that this was a change for the better. The students clearly settled into the process, and the much improved attendance rate was noted.

All this contributed to PBL becoming a part of the diploma programme, which reached its end in December 1999. The whole process and the information gained have been highly valued in terms of informing the 'new' programme. If a similar opportunity arises, carrying out a pilot study is highly recommended.

Finance

There are cost implications to this that include, for example, lecturer time, print room costs, and room usage. The author and her colleague have been particularly fortunate in that much of this work has been supported by winning a teaching fellowship – an internal university award that funds replacement teaching – 2 years running. On that note, it is worth mentioning that some lecturers will be reluctant to become facilitators because of the time taken. However, in our experience, the minimum time taken with each group is 2 hours per week. The commitment lies in the weekly session, the remaining time perhaps being taken up by acting as a resource person. It can be lecturer intensive, as, in our case, each module requires a minimum of 12 facilitators; as each PBL module comes 'on line' and runs each semester, the staff requirements can thus be daunting. To prepare for this, facilitators currently take two groups each, usually from different modules. In the future, this may need to be increased to taking two groups per module and scheduling group sessions whereby a number of groups are timetabled for one room, rather than the wider group all having their individual PBL session at the same time.

The future

The future of PBL in our school is exciting and sometimes a little frightening. Our motto is 'Share the Experience', and we firmly believe in this. This starts at PBL group level with students talking about life experiences and their contributions to packages, through to our networking via conference papers, journal articles and accessing the Internet. We can only develop by sharing information, and we have to date been involved in talking to people from other institutions. This opportunity is invaluable for sharing ideas, viewing documentation and, when possible, talking to students.

In June 1998, we hosted a PBL in Nursing conference. This was well received, being attended by approximately 45 delegates, who were able to make this an interactive conference rather than one in which people only presented their work. It was also pleasing to welcome colleagues from both ends of the UK, especially when financial support for attending conferences is becoming more difficult to obtain. The evaluations were most helpful, the highlight for most of the delegates being the opportunity to talk to students in an informal atmosphere over lunch.

Spreading the word includes writing for journals, and while our research activity has to date been minimal, articles have appeared in *Nursing Times* (Gibbon, 1998) and *PROBE*, the Australian PBL Network journal (Gibbon and Wall, 1998).

We presented our early forays into PBL at the Nurse Education Tomorrow Conference in Durham 1997, which again allowed welcome opportunities for discussion with colleagues. The development of the PBL modules has meant that more and more staff are involved in the process, and we can now start looking to the future and how the programme can proceed. Some ideas are already starting to become reality:

- Funds have become available from a university trust fund to develop teaching innovations. Toward this end, a project has been commenced on creating a videotape learning package. This will take the form of one of the current paper packages. A script has been written by a colleague who has experience of writing plays for radio, and another colleague, with extensive experience in the theatre, is masterminding the production with professional actors.

- Leading on from this project is the intention to put supplementary packs on to the Liverpool John Moores University Network. Students will be able to access further information related to their packs using guiding icons. There is a great deal of support for this notion, and the development will include representatives from all user groups.

- Some packs will need to continue as paper packages, a future idea being to experiment with an unfolding pack that will take the students through the whole of one module, that is, 12 teaching weeks. The student may, for example, take on the role of a community nurse working with a family for whom there are a number of issues apparent. Alternatively, the student may be the nurse in charge of a ward, dealing with patient situations, a staff member with a drink problem, and issues relating to catering, refuse disposal or missing drugs.

- The idea of a UK Network for PBL in Nursing, with a regular newsletter, was floated at the June 1998 conference.

- Work has already commenced on students' self-directed study skills. It is hoped to make this work a two-centre study that will allow scope for comparing and contrasting the skills that students bring with them on commencing a course, and then reviewing those skills on a regular basis.

- How a facilitator facilitates clearly varies from individual to individual. It is contended, however, that there are key skills required to make a success of the PBL process (cf. Chapter 6). There has been a great deal written about interpersonal skills, but an embryonic idea suggests that other or different skills may be required in PBL groups.

- The importance of clinical links can not be overstated. It has been recognised in this university that there is a need for an academic to work more closely with clinical staff in order to make the student experience more meaningful. This post entails 2 days per week clinical involvement, this being in addition to the requirement for lecturers to spend 20 per cent of their time in the clinical area. At the current time, four of these posts have been devised to cover the whole area used for clinical placements. However, these posts will provide an ideal opportunity to encourage the PBL and help students to make meaningful links between theory and practice.

- Leading on from these new roles, there will be scope for the development of PBL mentors and preceptors. The role of mentor is currently vague for preregistration students in our area, and using PBL will help to build that relationship. The role of preceptor may lie some way in the future, but the possibilities are there waiting to be explored.

- Evaluations from clinical staff will be vital to indicate how we proceed with PBL and whether we can encourage clinical staff to become facilitators.

The interest in PBL has always been present within other subject areas in the university. To encourage this interest, an internal conference across all disciplines was held in December 1998, whereby thoughts and ideas relating to PBL were discussed. The conference was attended by 40 delegates and stimulated an interactive day, with requests for similar ventures. The work on PBL in nursing is clearly creating a great deal of interest.

Conclusion

Implementing PBL into a preregistration nursing programme has presented the School of Health with many challenges. Some of these challenges have been overcome, and more, for example the staff required as facilitators, have yet to be faced. The school, like any school offering nursing programmes, is dynamic. PBL can offer that oasis of calm as a commitment to PBL is a regular, usually weekly, commitment to the students. Whether PBL is adopted as a whole philosophy or as a teaching and learning methodology, innovation is vital. There is a cautionary note, however, in that it is all too easy to become a PBL bore. Despite this, a quiet determination from all concerned that one will succeed will make it worthwhile. There is a great deal of satisfaction in using PBL, and also some frustration in terms of time expended, but positive evaluations from students, clinical and academic staff demonstrate that this is the right approach. In the words of Donald Woods (1994, Chapter 10, p. 6):

> PBL is the richest learning environment you will probably encounter in your lifetime. Savour it and enjoy.

References

Alavi, C (1995) *Problem-based Learning in a Health Sciences Curriculum*, Routledge: London.

Biley, F (1998) Evaluating a Welsh Undergraduate Nursing Education PBL Programme: A Short Report, *PROBE*, **18**: 12–13.

Doring, A, Bramwell-Vial A and Bingham B (1995) Staff Comfort/Discomfort with Problem-based Learning. A Preliminary Study. *Nurse Education Today*, **15**: 263–6.

Gibbon, C (1998) Problem-based Learning: Giving Control to the Student, *Nursing Times Learning Curve*, **2**(4): 4–5.

Gibbon, C and Wall, C (1998) A Strategy for Introducing Problem-based Learning, *PROBE*, **19**: 17–18.

Gugliomeno, A (1977) Development of Self-directed Learning Readiness Scale. Doctoral Dissertation, University of Georgia, *Dissertations Abstracts International 1978*: **38**: 64–7.

Hengstberger-Sims, C and McMillan, M (1993) Problem-based Learning Packages: Considerations for Neophyte Package Writers, *Nurse Education Today*, **13**: 73–7.

John, C (1994) Nuances of Reflection, *Journal of Clinical Nursing*, **4**: 23–30.

McMillan, M and Dwyer, J (1989) Changing Times, Changing Paradigm, Part 2: The MacArthur Experience, *Nurse Education Today*, **9**: 93–9.

Woods, D (1994) *Problem-based Learning: How to Gain the Most From PBL*, Waterdown, Ontario: Donald Woods.

4

Introducing Enquiry-based Learning into Preregistration Nursing Programmes

Garth Long and Sue Grandis

Background

The School of Nursing and Midwifery at the University of Southampton introduced an EBL approach for all preregistration nursing and midwifery programmes at Diploma, Advanced Diploma and Bachelor level in September 1997. The selection of the EBL process followed a review and subsequent development of the curriculum, which recognised that students needed to develop a questioning approach to evidence-based practice early in their course. A variety of strategies were considered to enhance the need for enquiry and thus capitalise on students' natural thirst for knowledge. EBL captures the initial motivation and continuing need of individuals to learn, and, by permitting the exploration of the status of current knowledge on a wide range of issues relevant to healthcare, complements the notion of evidence-based practice with the ever-present need to review the rationale for assumed knowledge (ENB, 1998).

EBL seeks to develop skills in reflection, clinical reasoning and critical thinking. The approach is based on the exploration of concepts from practice, which are derived from authentic client experiences and presented as scenarios. Each scenario forms the basis of a learning module over a period of 4–6 weeks, which is called a nursing unit. Team-working, with students taking increasing responsibility for their own learning, is emphasised. The aims of EBL, and many of the skills developed, for example leadership, team-working, collaboration and self-reliance in learning and in practice, can be seen to be very similar to those of PBL.

The National Board for Nursing, Midwifery and Health Visiting for Scotland (1998) recommends that, in order to be prepared to work in the current (and future) healthcare climate, nursing and midwifery students will need to develop and use a wide range of key, or transferable, skills, including problem-setting and problem-solving strategies. The process of enquiry reaches broadly to encompass concept analysis, critical analysis, framing and reframing issues for exploration, reflection, negotiation, thinking and working creatively and flexibly. These skills will continue to develop through the individual's career. Lifelong learning characteristics are the hallmark of an EBL curriculum. Through effective programme-planning, students have every opportunity to develop and practise skills to become (ENB, 1994, p. 6):

- innovative in their practice
- **flexible** to changing demand
- **resourceful** in their methods of working
- able to work as **change agents**
- able to **share good practice** and knowledge
- **adaptable** to changing healthcare needs
- challenging and **creative** in their practice
- **self-reliant** in their way of working
- **responsible and accountable** for their work.

The EBL group process is designed specifically to enhance each student's learning experience and to broaden and deepen the collective knowledge and understanding of all group members. Students are encouraged to use their personal well-established learning styles, to review their effectiveness and to consider how further to develop their ways of learning.

Developing the initiative

The School of Nursing and Midwifery had been working towards a whole-programme integrated EBL approach, building on the evolution of Project 2000 courses from the traditional programmes. Adult, Child, Mental Health, Learning Disability and Midwifery teachers were geographically close at the time of curriculum review, this proximity contributing to the feasibility of joint planning. Combined experiences were mutually beneficial. Potential opportunities for shared planning had clear benefits of time-saving, for example in developing study packs and resources. Increasing shared learning opportunities would also enhance the diversity and richness of experience across all these fields. Strong working partnerships were forged, and, in retrospect, it is fortunate that this opportunity was capitalised upon as the school has since expanded rapidly from one site working with two Trusts, to several sites and many Trusts.

Introducing clinical practice early in the programme had been well established and was deemed to be an essential ingredient to complement an EBL approach. Adjustments were made to capitalise on this by further increasing the amount of practice earlier in the programme. In each 4-week nursing unit, 2 weeks are spent in practice. The same placement is accessed across a number of nursing units in a semester, giving at least 20 days' assessed experience in each placement. The first placement is field specific, providing the 'picture on the box' so that students have an early view of what is expected of them and can verify the relevance of their learning. This being field specific from the outset is believed to enable students to achieve a strong early identity and engagement with their particular branch of nursing, helping them to see the relevance of common and shared learning opportunities, as well as increasing motivation. Local needs also influenced the retention of strategies to develop reflective practice. Local public health issues and the resulting needs were reviewed. Local Trusts expected value for money and competent practitioners. Recognising nursing as the central focus, valuing appropriate expertise and producing a curriculum that is educationally sound, one which motivates students to engage with the process of learning, are all cornerstones of the EBL approach.

A core curriculum group (CCG) was convened, which, to ensure ownership of the new programmes, included subject specialists, community teachers and local community and acute NHS Trusts representatives. It became obvious early in the group's life that there were differing agendas. There were debates over the philosophy and what should take precedence, for example nursing specialties, subjects, community versus hospital, health versus illness and degree versus diploma. An independent educational consultant as a CCG member proved invaluable in resolving these tensions. Midwifery had its own CCG, although there was representation across both groups. The experience of small-group facilitation for reflective practice in each of the fields in the existing programmes was influential in shaping the new curriculum. Facilitators for the initial EBL groups had all been reflective group facilitators. This experience also helped in making pragmatic decisions about group size, group mix, booking space and frequency of group meetings.

The work of the CCG was supported by field-specific planning groups (branches plus midwifery), which included practitioners, students, consumers and teachers, who all worked to the same broad framework as the CCG. The school hosted presentations about PBL that confirmed for the CCG that, even though PBL had a lot to offer, our programmes would also use a variety of other teaching and learning strategies. To verify these decisions, the Director of Curriculum and the EBL Co-ordinator attended an international PBL conference in Canada, hosted by McMaster University. In addition to learning from the presentations, they met individuals already involved in PBL from all over the world – colleagues from Canada, the USA and Australia who were particularly helpful in endorsing our thinking on PBL. They thus returned to the UK with a clearer strategy of how to take the development forward (McMaster University, 1996).

The most important aspect of the change process was the need to ensure that everyone involved in programme delivery would understand the philosophy, support it, own it and develop it. This was essential as there was a risk that teachers who did not agree with a particular philosophy, or felt threatened by it, might employ strategies which were counter-productive to this new way of working, and might undermine the programme aims (cf. Chapter 2). There are also areas for potential misunderstanding. For example, when phrases such as 'adult learning' and 'working in small groups' are used, some teachers may feel that they are already engaged in these processes and do not appreciate how different the strategy will be when using EBL as an integrated, whole-programme approach. Protagonists proved beneficial as, when disagreements arose, discussion often resulted in a clearer rationale for all the plans being progressed. Others identified gaps or put forward new arguments that helped to develop further ideas or overcome shortfalls. Through this process, programmes became yet more robust.

From the outset, it was realised that if a radically different approach were to be taken in educating nursing and midwifery students, a more significant input would be required from service colleagues. It was essential to ensure that the new curriculum would develop the knowledge, skills and attitudes needed locally by the newly qualified practitioners. This involved keeping clinical staff informed and included, in particular, listening, valuing and giving credit to their contributions.

A consultation group that represented all the main interest groups and stakeholders, including users and clinical staff, was established. More then 70 people were involved, and it became a useful sounding board for ideas and developments. Although members regularly responded to drafts sent for comment, face-to-face meetings were often poorly attended because of competing clinical demands. A battery of information-giving activities regularly targeted different interest groups. These included a newsletter directed at clinical staff, 'roadshow' presentations on different sites where people could come and ask questions, presentations to clinical managers, information sessions for existing students, and informal information-giving by link teachers in their day-to-day support of the learning environment. No single activity was deemed to be more important than another. It was acknowledged that the new curriculum would introduce a radically different model, yet it was quickly seen by clinical staff to have face validity. Information that staff required in order to become familiar with the approach needed to be repeated several times in different formats and different venues, each package addressing different needs. Specific updating workshops were provided for clinical staff who were already acting as student clinical assessors. Existing courses for preparing assessors were adapted to include experience of the EBL process for the course participants.

Keeping clinical staff involved

Although the motivation and commitment of clinical staff and managers were high, as stated they found difficulty in finding the time to attend regular meetings. Students enjoyed the challenge and contributed fully to the process. They were eager to find ways of improving upon their own learning experiences, being keen to promote more student autonomy and choice, while recognising the difficulties in bringing about change in some areas because of limited resources. To ensure an involved representation of all groups, the CCG, which was intentionally restricted to a small number of educationalists, clinical staff and students, met weekly. This group was strategic, focusing on the philosophy and processes needed to deliver the EBL curriculum. It also needed to ensure that, although a field-specific approach would be maintained from the outset, requirements for a CFP would be met and opportunities for integration and shared learning capitalised upon. There were also four field-planning groups that looked more specifically and in more depth at the branch-specific curriculum needs from the beginning of CFP to the end of each branch. Each group represented the interests of stakeholders, and the field groups ensured that the views of users were acknowledged. Since validation, the day-to-day responsibility for the programme has now shifted to the preregistration course management team, and subgroups continuing to represent the specific field interests.

Listening and giving credit

As anticipated, there was a degree of resistance to some of the proposals. It was essential, therefore, that all contributors perceived that they were listened to and had their views acknowledged. This did not necessarily mean that changes were always made to accommodate views that were at odds with the majority. At times, it was difficult to find the evidence to counter individual challenges as the probable outcomes of some of the curriculum approaches were unknown or had never been tested in a similar context. As well as the philosophical debates mentioned above, there were ongoing discussions about a range of issues. These included specialist versus generalist EBL facilitation, freedom to learn through a range of resources or reliance on main hall compulsory lectures, and monitored attendance or open access and choice.

A major concern was whether students would be able to demonstrate depth as well as breadth in achieving outcomes (cf. Chapter 2). A research study into the outcome competences for students graduating from the existing curriculum had been set up in partnership between the school and the two local purchasers. Although not directly related to the new developments, this reinforced the spirit of collaboration in relation to curriculum development and evaluation (O'Connor *et al.*, 1998).

Ongoing local evaluation findings relating to existing programmes were considered as part of the curriculum development process. Clinical staff and students were also involved in a comprehensive review of the school's Assessment of Practice scheme. This enabled the clinical staff to take a lead in developing a new practice assessment tool, one that they would see as being valid and reliable, and one that would meet their needs. Through this initiative, clinical staff were able to own and feel confident in introducing these new instruments.

Designing the curriculum

As practice is central to the EBL curriculum, the learning packages in the nursing units had to reflect this. Fifty per cent of the programmes comprise nursing practice starting in the first month of the nursing programmes. From the first week, students begin to develop practical confidence in the skills centre giving hands-on care such as moving and handling, nursing observations and hygiene needs, while exploring such concepts as touch, communication, trust and gender issues arising from the EBL scenarios.

There is increasing evidence that an appropriate questioning approach, developed by students using EBL, contributes to conscious decisions to review and change practice (Boud and Feletti, 1997). On completion of the programme, the emerging practitioner should possess the self-confidence and readiness to be adaptable, accountable and effective in liaison with others to change practice. Discussing and reflecting on practice in EBL group sessions is a valuable part of this process. Acknowledging ground rules of confidentiality, students describe events from practice experience and link these to the underpinning theory. Initially, only description is offered, but as confidence in making judgements about practice grows within the group, students explore and analyse situations in detail. Using a reflective cycle and critical analysis framework, students are encouraged to consider satisfying, uncomfortable and distressing situations. Behaviours, joys, sadness and many other feelings can be recounted with clarity, openness and honesty. Comments written by the student and the clinical assessor in the practice documentation endorse these experiences. In the student's portfolio of learning, further details of specific incidents are developed into a more comprehensive reflective account.

Learning needs and opportunities needed to be packaged in a way that enhanced the EBL approach. Creating such packages was an interesting challenge as students' motivation to enquire and learn should be naturally stimulated rather than manipulated. Learning outcomes for the packages needed to relate to both programme and year goals in order to ensure that learning, although under student control, met the needs of the course, that is, demonstrated the centrality of nursing practice.

Outcomes identified for programmes cannot be viewed as exclusive as concept generation is not an exact science, the nature of a concept clearly being dynamic. Within each nursing unit, students have the opportunity to explore concepts that they perceive as being relevant. The list of concepts important to nursing, for example caring, health, roles and attitudes, is extensive. Further concepts derive from learning, for example self as a learner, enquiry and evidence. Others, such as interpersonal skills, altered communication and working collaboratively, relate to communication. Learning opportunities were designed around such concepts and content.

Programme content draws on the themes of nursing, health, biological sciences, pharmacology, first aid, health and safety, ethics, law, sociology and social policy, psychology, management and communication. Topic areas such as health education, care-planning, infection control and chronic illness are included. A review of which specific conditions to include, for example diabetes, and asthma, was undertaken to ensure validity and relevance in relation to local health profiles (WHO, 1993); each nursing unit focuses on one or more health or disease processes.

An integrated approach was achieved by allowing the learning content to arise from within each scenario. This provides the initial stimulus required to motivate students to engage in broad and deep learning (cf. Chapters 1, 2 and 8). Scenarios, created from the real health experiences of clients or patients, are devised by teachers with specific clinical or research interest in the topic, in liaison with community and clinical practitioners. Different media are used to present scenarios; there may be a paper introduction to a client, or a snippet of a video or audiotape of a nurse's hand-over. The school had considerable experience of using the reflective cycle and wanted to retain this. Elements of the problem-solving and reflective cycles were incorporated into the Southampton process – a model of EBL that the students follow to acquire the necessary learning to meet specified outcomes.

The Southampton process

Guided by the student chair and supported by the facilitator, students continuously check their understanding of the scenario. Clarity with regard to the context is established with guidance from the facilitator if required. The group then brainstorms issues that arise directly from the scenario, and the scribe records these on a flipchart or a board. The Facilitator's Guide provides more information, for example social details, health history and complementary nursing notes such as charts, care plans and investigation results, which can be accessed by students at the discretion of the facilitator as the scenario unfolds. The students are encouraged to provide a rationale for requesting the further details. It is essential that students work with materials incrementally rather than being given the whole scenario at once. To avoid the risk of omitting important areas for enquiry and preventing students going down 'blind alleys', the facilitator guides students so that they can focus more deeply on particular aspects. Questions are framed, and as individuals in the group find answers, they share their information. Further learning needs are agreed as questions are refined and prioritised. The nature of each question will depend on issues such as the learning outcomes for the nursing unit, as well as group/personal interests and learning needs. The facilitator gives guidance according to the stage reached in the programme, but, as long as specified outcomes are achieved, exploring other relevant issues is not discouraged.

The EBL group affords students opportunities to check out the validity of their perceived learning needs and their understanding of what they are learning, and to gauge the required depth of learning by picking up on cues offered by other group members. The facilitator is proactive in judging whether a considered intervention will inhibit or enhance the group process, and ensures that opportunities are not missed. Students more readily give and seek feedback in this encouraging, supportive working atmosphere, which is created by partnership between the facilitator and each student, working to the group's ground rules.

Seeking answers to questions is managed in a variety of ways. Each nursing unit lasts approximately 4–6 weeks and includes a mixture of clinical practice, theory, course work and, during the foundation programme, community time. The group reviews the planned timetable of learning opportunities, which includes a number of fixed resource sessions. These may include lectures, on for example biological science, sociology or psychology, skills centre sessions and, possibly, communication workshops. Many of these will make use of linked multimedia opportunities. Further concurrent sessions offer interesting learning experiences for a smaller number of students, for example mixed group workshops, tutorials and presentations by practitioners, users and clients sharing their experiences. Individuals elect to represent their group at these sessions and to put the group's questions. An introductory list of additional resources is suggested in the Nursing Unit Student Guide, including references (journals, indicative textbooks, government reports and local policy documents) and other materials – videos, CD-ROMs, websites, novels and poems, for example.

Questions are prioritised according to the opportunities available before the next EBL group meeting. If practice-based experience is to follow immediately, specific practice-related questions are reviewed and shared between the group. The students may then take some of these questions to their placements and discuss them with their clinical assessors. For example, in the first nursing unit, students may seek answers to the questions 'What is caring?' and 'What are the behaviours that demonstrate a caring attitude?' Each student in the group has a different placement, so the variety of experiences, which contributes to their early learning, is immense.

Community-related questions are taken to community discussion groups that meet during the foundation programme. As each nursing unit is planned with community teachers, this ensures that learning opportunities arise from and complement the scenario. Apart from planned sessions and library resources, students are also encouraged to network and access people and places, using these as resources related to the chosen topics. Students become very resourceful in discovering useful contacts, and further develop their interpersonal and communication skills, including time management and negotiation. At the following EBL group meeting, each student provides feedback about the community experience. The group shares this information and uses it to meet its learning outcomes.

Most of the nursing unit information, including timetables and concept lists, is located on the school web pages and is therefore accessible to students and staff. Subject co-ordinators (for themes such as psychology, sociology, health and safety at work, and communication) identify key content for the lectures and suggest additional multimedia resources. Links from these web pages to other resources are continually being developed.

In the foundation programme, nursing units include shared learning opportunities to service the needs of all the field-specific groups. Later, learning packs are used that target field-specific content and promote the development of, for example, team-working, communication and information-giving skills. Conference days contribute to shared learning. By working in partnership with other group members and the facilitator, students exercise a choice regarding learning methods. Signposts for each unit of learning (for example, learning outcomes) help students to remain focused as they decide what additional personal or group outcomes they wish to pursue, whether to work individually or collectively, and when and where.

The EBL group's field-specific facilitator is the student's academic tutor and performs essential roles in complementing and supporting the integrated approach to learning.

The student experience

The EBL curriculum framework supports the expectation that students will meet weekly in their EBL groups with their facilitator and, less frequently, in non-facilitated meetings. Group dynamics may be affected by various aspects and must be managed. The age range may be wide, life experiences vary considerably, and, in most groups, there will be both male and female students with diverse backgrounds, academic levels and cultures. Students learn to respect and value each member of the group and the contribution that each makes, whatever their age, gender, ability or culture. This diverse mix of people is reflected in healthcare settings among clients, patients, relatives, visitors, colleagues and multidisciplinary team members, so students have valuable opportunities within the EBL group to practise skills related to managing themselves and others in the world of healthcare. Students take it in turns to take on the roles of chair and scribe, which further enhances learning in a group. Listening, formulating and asking questions appropriately, challenging each other and managing such challenges confidently are skills learnt through effective group process.

Group-working may initially be an uncomfortable experience. There may be irritation or anger, for example at constant lateness or a lack of contribution by some members, inappropriate language, verbal aggression, frustration or embarrassment, while some students remain quiet, hoping that others will sort out the difficulties. Through careful and thoughtful interventions, the facilitator manages the group; this may, for example, include using humour or reframing the problem in order to help the group move on. These experiences contribute to the development of a wide range of behaviours, including assertiveness, challenging appropriately, self-awareness, diplomacy and negotiation.

The regular expectation placed on students to present to their peers using a range of approaches reinforces group cohesion and increases confidence. From the beginning, students are encouraged to own previous experiences and capitalise on them, and they quickly learn from each other to use a range of strategies to convey information. Verbal presentations are complemented by flipcharts, acetates, slides, some producing videos. Role-play is used in some groups, the facilitator being given a specific part and being guided by the student on how to manage the role. There is little room in the process for the facilitator to impose a method of working on the group. Group members may value guidance, especially where this is invited, but they may also reject it. Students readily learn from each other and develop confidence to try different ideas, becoming innovative and adaptable.

Working relationships develop. Students quickly learn to give and receive compliments, plan and share the workload equitably, manage a personal workload and become accountable. A sense of increasing self-reliance and responsibility also contributes towards the early emergence of leadership qualities.

The need for safety in a group is often highlighted in education in order for the group to support its members in learning. However, the group can also initially be perceived as powerful and threatening, especially to students new to the experience of learning in a group, so the process needs to be managed from the beginning and constantly encouraged. Others may be reticent, although willing, and there have been some very pleasing moments when, after some time, students are able to value how much they have developed through the process. Publicity materials must be explicit about the EBL method and the implications for learning in such a climate. Group-working is not an easy option and is not natural to most people, although most candidates will say that they enjoy group-work. The method does not suit everyone, and persistent negative attitudes and behaviour can disrupt group processes. Selecting students with the potential to benefit from and succeed in such an environment is essential.

The skills of personal reflection are developed through discussion with group members and the academic tutor, practice experience, academic assignments and contributions to their portfolio of learning. Some students also keep a reflective diary. It is through this supportive group process that students have every opportunity to be open and honest about areas in need of development and find ways of enhancing and capitalising on their natural skills and talents. The beginnings of key and transferable skills can be seen to develop through EBL. These skills are essential if the individual is to practise effectively in a world of multidisciplinary and multi-agency healthcare working.

Reflection

The first year of implementation was characterised by considerable energy and enthusiasm, both from teachers who were keen to have the opportunity to lead from the front and to teach nursing, and from students who were very motivated by exploring scenarios that were taken from real client experiences. This, together with early clinical practice and community activities, meant that students were able to identify and experience nursing – something that all had entered the course to do. Most students were quick to engage with the principles of EBL although facilitation styles differed considerably between the groups. This caused some initial concern to those who would have felt more secure had everyone been taking the same approach, but the students did not seem to mind and quickly identified with the style of their facilitator.

Some students were less satisfied, some found the EBL process alien to and incompatible with their preferred learning style, and some had come from a school or college where the curriculum had been delivered in a highly structured way. Many of these students had been recruited to the programme prior to the school's taking the decision to introduce the principles of EBL on the interview day. On reflection, this was one of the most important aspects of all. By carrying out a short EBL activity as a group, applicants were introduced to the processes of enquiry. This included group processes, and the role of scribe and chair, which helped them to recognise the need to take responsibility for each other as well as themselves. Candidates were left in no doubt as to what was to be expected of them, and the few who felt unable to accept the challenge went elsewhere.

Central to the development and implementation of EBL has been a planned and phased programme of staff development, facilitator preparation and updating. This has encompassed a range of activities that have included all staff involved with the programme. A continuing programme of training has enabled staff to develop email and computer skills. Although electronic resources were, and still are, used as the main information channel for providing information to the school's staff, a range of other methods were employed, including staff meetings, the school's internal 'news sheet' and a constantly updated information file placed in staff rooms. Since that time, a range of additional communication channels have become established to support staff, provide information and deal with queries. These are in addition to the school's formal processes required for evaluation and curriculum development.

The success of any initiative undoubtedly lies in commitment from the top, in terms of both resources and voicing that support publicly whenever the opportunity presents itself. This was essential in the development of a scheme that might initially be seen as high cost and high risk. There were four key players who supported the initiative in various ways and contributed to its successful implementation:

- *Educational purchasers.* Not long after the successful validation of the programme, the school engaged in competitive tendering, and as a result, a sizeable commission for the provision of pre- and postregistration nursing education materialised. The purchasers were clearly attracted by both the process of EBL, the flexibility of delivery and outcomes that can be achieved through this curriculum model. The philosophy that underpins EBL, which stimulates enquiry, problem-solving, critical thinking and reflection, is one that identifies with health service priorities, including the need to provide evidence-based healthcare through a team approach.

- *Statutory bodies.* A supportive and involved ENB Officer provided essential encouragement during programme-planning and implementation.

- *The university.* The university supported the major developments and innovations that the school was committed to pursuing. The university was asked to approve structures and processes that were sometimes quite alien to more traditional university programmes. The university also supported the development through to conjoint validation.

- *The School of Nursing.* The success of the scheme also has relied heavily on the continuing involvement of and close liaison with library services, from the outset of planning to ongoing delivery of the programme. It also provides students with access to course information, student notes, search facilities and

Internet access. The most important aspect was, however, the total commitment by the head of the school to fund and resource this curriculum approach. Such commitment from the top is paramount to success.

Facing the challenge

There were, however, difficulties to be overcome. Some were practical issues. Early in the course, some students were unable to gain access to the computer system because of delays in registration. Some subject co-ordinators had been more proactive than others in ensuring that student notes and other resources were available in good time and displayed on the Web pages. Although many of the facilitators were well experienced in running groups, some found some of the group dynamics challenging. In addition, some students, unused to the potential freedom of EBL, became manipulative and challenged group norms. In many cases, the groups dealt with the problem internally, but on occasions facilitators had to intervene. As group identity has become stronger and expectations made explicit, students find difficulty in not adhering to group rules.

The delivery of the course relies heavily on those educationalists who are EBL facilitators, the cohort co-ordinators and those in secretarial and administrative roles. It is therefore imperative to involve all staff in ongoing presentations and information sessions to ensure that we continue to learn from the experience.

That experience has, to date, been positive, and we believe that the programme will produce practitioners who, in addition to possessing the knowledge to practise competently, have the ability to respond flexibly and imaginatively to the unexpected, and who own the need to continually enquire and update themselves. These practitioners will be rooted in practice and will continue to learn from and in practice, while contributing to the development of the body of nursing knowledge. We remain firm in our conviction that the Southampton EBL programme goes a long way towards addressing the challenges facing the profession.

References

Boud, D and Feletti, G I (eds) (1997) *The Challenge of Problem-based Learning*, (2nd edn), London: Kogan Page.

English National Board for Nursing, Midwifery and Health Visiting (1994) *Creating Lifelong Learners – Partnerships for Care*, London: ENB.

English National Board for Nursing, Midwifery and Health Visiting (1998) D*evelopments in the Use of an Evidence and/or Enquiry Based Approach in Nursing, Midwifery and Health Visiting Programmes of Education*, http://www.enb.org.uk/evidpub.htm.

McMaster University (1996) *BScN Handbook*. Hamilton, Ontario.

National Board for Nursing, Midwifery and Health Visiting for Scotland (1998) *Information Base on Arrangements which Support the Development of Clinical Practice in Pre-registration Nursing Programmes in Scotland*, Edinburgh: NBS.

O'Connor, S, Pearce, J, Smith, R, Vogeli, D and Walton, P (1998) Monitoring the Quality of Pre-Registration Education: Final Report. A Joint Research Project by the Southampton University Hospital, NHS Trust and Community Health Services NHS Trust, Southampton: University of Southampton School of Nursing and Midwifery.

World Health Organisation (1993) *Increasing the Relevance of Education for Health Professions,* Report of a WHO Study Group on Problem-solving Education for the Health Professionals, Technical Report Series No. 838, Geneva: WHO.

5

Problem-based Learning in Midwifery

Joyce Wise

Introduction

In the early 1990's, in response to the Winterton report (House of Commons Health Committee 1992), the Department of Health (DoH) set up an Expert Maternity Group, chaired by Baroness Cumberlege, Parliamentary Under Secretary of State for Health, to investigate the then current provision of maternity care within the NHS. In 1993, the findings were collated and a report, called *Changing Childbirth*, was produced (DoH, 1993). This report made a number of key recommendations that were intended to act as a catalyst to radically reform the maternity services provided in England. From a fragmented style of care provision that favoured organisations and staff, it was proposed that care should become woman centred and incorporate what subsequently became known as the 3 C's: Choice, Control and Continuity of Care for women. For effective service provision, it was identified in the report that midwives needed to utilise the full range of skills that they possessed on qualification. In this way, organisational systems, such as 'caseload holding', that would facilitate continuity of care by midwifes could be set up.

The implications of this proposed change for midwives in practice were, to say the least, significant. For those midwives who had worked in fragmented care systems for a number of years, the proposal raised a number of issues, for example the education needs that became apparent in order to help individual practitioners feel confident and competent to offer this style of care. Within the Isle of Wight Maternity Service, this issue was addressed through the production and use of a 'resource-based' educational package that was designed to help to prepare midwives for implementing a caseload-holding style of service delivery. The challenge was to meet a wide variety of learning needs that midwives identified and to facilitate change in practice using a PBL approach as a central feature of the education experience. This chapter describes the development, implementation and evaluation of this study pack, entitled Caseload Management in Midwifery Practice.

The project – setting the scene

In 1994, when this project began, the national picture of maternity service provision was one of diversity. Some maternity units still operated 'fragmented systems of care'. In these, women moved through the system meeting new teams of midwives in community and hospital, and if hospitalised, in areas specifically offering antenatal, labour and postnatal care. It is clear to see that women rarely experienced continuity of care within this approach; in fact, a documentation review demonstrated that one woman met up to 45 midwives during her contact with this type of maternity service (Wise, 1988). This may not even have been the worst-case scenario, and it was certainly not conducive to forming relationships. Other maternity units in the country, in response to growing discontent from women over a perceived lack of continuity of care, were either operating, or moving towards adopting, team systems of care. The team systems were designed to improve continuity of care by midwives, but took various shapes depending on local circumstances and need.

On the Isle of Wight, a fragmented system of care had been in operation until 1992, when, following a locally commissioned report on maternity service provision, a team system was eventually put in place, reflecting national trends (Wise, 1988). Two teams were created in the hospital, the midwives in each team caring for approximately 600 women a year. The groups of women came from specific geographical areas, and the hospital team was linked to the appropriate community-based midwives and GPs. Now, instead of women moving through the system, the intention was that they stayed with the same group of midwives throughout all their contacts with the service. Although to some extent this improved continuity of care, women were still meeting a lot of midwives. The presence of what were called 'core teams' in the antenatal clinic and labour suite, while of value, meant that midwives were still not able to develop all their skills in caring for women across the continuum of pregnancy to parenthood. With the publication of the *Changing Childbirth* report in 1993, it became apparent that an even more radical change was imminent. In order to implement the proposals, a significant education need was identified for midwives, who were still working in a semi-fragmented care environment.

A total of 65 midwives were employed by the Isle of Wight (NHS) Trust. Each came from different levels of preregistration preparation for practice and had a wide variety and length of post-qualification experience. They also differed in the level of cross-continuum care in which they were involved, and had expressed many and diverse personal learning needs. The more 'traditional' approaches to education, for example formal courses, statutory midwifery refresher courses or study day attendance, seemed inadequate to accommodate all of these aspects in an effective way. Formal courses could potentially have covered a wider range of learning needs in time, but they would clearly have been very expensive to resource in terms of both course fees and staff absence from the workplace. What could be included in a study day that would meet everyone's learning needs? Attendance at study days included varying degrees of participant involvement. To prepare midwives to practise more independently and autonomously, this approach was unlikely to establish the self-directed style of learning that would be necessary for caseload-holding practice.

The dilemma of how to prepare midwives for operating a new care system was the initial problem to solve. An education strategy was needed that was flexible enough to take into account the multiplicity of backgrounds and experience, but focused enough to ensure that the learning achieved was relevant to the needs of each midwife. It also needed to be manageable in practical terms, those of structure and delivery, and financially. A review of the literature available at that time yielded very little in the way of suggestions on how to approach this specific task. Even in 1995, Stimson (1995) identified only a traditional programme of study days and courses as an integral part of the change process in the new system of care being developed in her area. She did not offer any detail on the focus or content of this study, or on the relevance of this input to the new working structures. A new and innovative approach had to be devised that specifically focused on preparation for caseload-holding.

The starting point in addressing this issue was to consider exactly what was required in practical terms. In essence, midwives needed to direct their own learning in a way that mirrored the work patterns they would be required to adopt. A form of open/distance learning seemed to be the most obvious and flexible solution. An adult learning approach was considered essential (Rogers, 1989), and a PBL component was eventually developed as an integral feature. According to Garbett (1996), this enables students to be creative and analytical, which, in conjunction with decision-making skills, is an essential element of caseload management. This was a novel approach to learning at that time, when midwives were predominantly used to the traditional forms of education already mentioned. PBL was not a central aspect of curriculum design in either preregistration or postregistration midwifery courses in the early 1990s, although it may well have been used as a teaching strategy in individual sessions. This has currently changed a little, some entire midwifery programmes of study now being built around a PBL framework. At the time, this project, developed though this approach to learning, was to some extent breaking new ground.

Development

The task of reviewing the midwifery service and formulating a plan for change in response to the *Changing Childbirth* report was taken on by a specially convened review group. This group was set up by the midwifery managers and included a number of people representing different areas of the service. Those involved were service managers, supervisors of midwives, clinical midwives from each team and myself from the University of Portsmouth in my role as midwifery link tutor. Medical colleagues were also invited to participate. The focus of the review group's work was to assess service provision as it was offered at that time against the 10 key indicators of successful change identified in the report (DoH, 1993, p.70) (Figure 5.1). It was in this forum, and on the basis of these indicators, that the main education issues for the midwives became apparent and the problems of how to address them were discussed.

- All women should be entitled to carry their own notes.
- Every woman should know one midwife who ensures continuity of her midwifery care – the named midwife.
- At least 30 per cent of women should have the midwife as the lead professional.
- Every woman should know the lead professional who has a key role in the planning and provision of her care.
- At least 75 per cent of women should *know* the person who cares for them during their delivery.
- Midwives should have direct access to some beds in all maternity units.
- At least 30 per cent of women delivered in a maternity unit should be admitted under the management of the midwife.
- The total number of antenatal visits for women with uncomplicated pregnancies should have been reviewed in the light of available evidence and the Royal College of Obstetricians and Gynaecologists' Guidelines.
- All frontline ambulances should have a paramedic able to support the midwife who needs to transfer a woman to hospital in an emergency.
- All women should have access to information about the services available in their locality.

Figure 5.1   Ten key indicators of success (DoH, 1993, p. 70)

Once the idea for a flexible-content study pack was agreed by the group, it was then necessary to seek approval and support from higher-level service managers and the NHS Trust to carry the idea forward. This was given wholeheartedly, and the project was welcomed as an innovative and useful way to progress. It became my task to begin work on the project. The first step was to carry out a more formal and widespread consultation with

the midwives regarding their perceived learning needs in relation to implementing change. Baseline information had already
been gathered in a questionnaire sent to all staff when the team
system had been introduced a couple of years earlier. This was
now updated as appropriate. The diversity of learning needs was
brought sharply into focus by this exercise. It was also clear from
the beginning that it was essential to work *with* the midwives on
this project rather than to offer an imposed strategy. In this way,
a sense of ownership could develop that was likely to increase
its chance of success, which is facilitated by PBL.

What should the study pack look like? In practical terms,
midwives needed to be able to assess and plan care from the
first antenatal visit through to 28 days post-delivery. This was not
happening in the existing organisational structure. Although
midwives were prepared for a full role on qualification, within a
fragmented system of care or even in team systems, many went
on to develop skills in only one specific part of practice. Also
'shared care' between hospital, community, midwifery and
medical colleagues meant that few, if any, midwives in the service
were taking full responsibility for all decisions related to care
management. To meet the requirements of undertaking a 'lead
professional' role, as identified in the indicators of success, this
factor would be required for change to be implemented successfully (DoH, 1993). In addition to these aspects, midwives needed
to be able to identify their own learning needs within practice
situations and take steps to address these in flexible and creative
ways. Accessing and utilising various reference sources was a
crucial part of this process and was promoted through the use
of PBL. The ability to reflect on practice and the establishment
of a principle of lifelong learning also needed to be developed.

The ultimate intention was to enable midwives to gain confidence in their own knowledge base and decision-making skills,
and to feel able to justify these decisions in a caseload management style of care. These factors became the underpinning
elements when the format of the study pack was decided, and
underlines another reason for using a PBL approach. The need
to assess and plan care from the first antenatal visit meant that
the starting point for the study pack became the creation of a
'booking history' for an individual (fictitious) woman. This would
act as a trigger for the whole strategy. From this booking history,

a *simulation* exercise over the continuum of care could be carried out with midwives clarifying need, problem-solving and justifying their main care decisions for each stage (cf. Chapter 2). Benner (1984) argues that undertaking simulation exercises is beneficial to practitioners as it enables them to develop confidence in their own decision-making skills. This was particularly important to achieve, and simulation exercises would also give midwives the opportunity to consolidate essential aspects of their role before change took place. Other reasons for undertaking a simulation exercise rather than using real cases were identified as (Wise, 1996):

- Avoiding the potential for breaking aspects of confidentiality within a small community.
- Allowing a freedom of expression in planning that might be constrained if the actual case were remembered.
- Enabling the midwife to plan for a wider variety of complicated cases than might be accessed from recent case notes.
- Helping individual midwives to become involved in the development process of their scenario, which should invoke a sense of ownership and allow them to follow their own learning needs.

The initial aims and learning outcomes of the study pack overall were becoming clearer and more focused.

Aims

- To enable midwives to enhance skills, knowledge and strategies for the management of a client caseload extending from the confirmation of pregnancy until 28 days postpartum.
- To facilitate the further development of the skills needed for self-directed, lifelong learning.

Learning outcomes

On completion of the package, the practitioner would have had the opportunity to:

- Identify, physical, social, psychological, spiritual and cultural factors within a midwifery case scenario.
- Examine and evaluate the available information, literature and research evidence in a range of selected areas, with a demonstration of the application of this knowledge via the development of a plan for individualised care.
- Demonstrate the ability to exercise professional judgement and argue coherently and rationally for decisions related to immediate and continuing care in pregnancy, labour and the puerperium.
- Analyse the interrelationship between the midwife and other health professionals in providing safe and effective maternity care.
- Analyse the extent of personal learning through an effective reflection strategy.

These learning outcomes have recently been modified to reflect the variety of uses to which the study pack has subsequently been put. At the start of the project, however, these were the learning outcomes expected, and the study pack content was designed to try to achieve them.

It was agreed that, for ease of development, the study pack would be created in discrete but conceptually linked sections. The package comprised sections each with its own specific aims, learning outcomes and sets of activities:

1. Antenatal first visit
2. Antenatal care through pregnancy:
   – booking – 24 weeks' gestation
   – 24 weeks' – onset of labour
3. Care in labour
4. Postnatal care of mother, baby and family up to 28 days post-delivery
5. Clinical practice links.

As the essential underpinning element, section 1 was completed first. The main task for the compiler was to generate a wide variety of booking scenarios covering as large a range of potential learning needs as possible, which would form the triggers for learning. This was seen as a crucial achievement if all 65 midwives were to have the opportunity to work on their own individual case study at their own pace. What seemed like a good idea to begin with quickly became a daunting task, and the idea was almost abandoned. The time it would take to sit and write this number of booking histories seemed prohibitive, but a stroke of good fortune helped to solve this problem. At the same time as this part of the project was being considered, late 1994 to early 1995, the maternity unit was planning to introduce a new computerised information system. This system used a program for record-keeping in pregnancy, labour and the postnatal period that was designed to standardise the way in which data were collected and retrieved. The opportunity to 'test' the system before it went into full-time use was too good to miss.

With the assistance of a midwife colleague, seconded to oversee the introduction of the computer system into practice, a total of 65 fictional history sheets was created. This took a fraction of the time it would have taken to complete the same job by hand. A variety of demographic, midwifery and obstetric situations were included, covering as many aspects as we and the computer system could come up with. We were convinced that we would be able to offer a scenario that could effectively trigger whatever learning needs a midwife expressed. Besides the time factor, a second advantage of this approach was that the study pack would use an information format mirroring the one used in practice. In this way, it was hoped that the simulated scenario would seem more 'real' and familiar.

Once the booking history scenarios were produced, the next stage was to introduce a 'guided study' element to the pack to give it structure. A series of activities were included that were based around the history sheet and the information it contained. One of the main elements was a process of assessing and planning care that would need to be undertaken by all midwives managing caseloads. A review of the scenario details would lead to an assessment of need and a framing of potential 'problems'. These problems were dual faceted: the primary focus would be related to the woman and her situation, and the secondary focus to problems that the midwife identified in relation to her or his own needs in order to successfully undertake this task. The plan of care could be produced in any format, but midwives would be guided to consider a range of aspects for the individual and her family, including:

- The significant factors identified from the history.
- Observations/examinations to be made.
- Tests/assessments to be offered for establishing maternal and fetal wellbeing.
- The focus of midwifery care at this visit.
- Options for the place of birth.
- Health professionals to be involved in care.
- Who was best placed to carry out the lead professional role.

A justification for these decisions was to be offered.

The assessment/planning process was further guided by the inclusion of a model of midwifery care that was developed in response to the proposed changes. This would provide a common framework within which to work – at a general level. To broaden thinking on issues related to the organisation and content of this first meeting between the woman and the midwife, a number of recommended readings were included. Only the reference was given for the readings, in order to encourage midwives to access the literature themselves, thus facilitating their library skills.

Another central element was the task of identifying one issue or area of practice, generated from the assessment/planning process, to study in more depth. As well as allowing knowledge development, this would enhance the skills of accessing information from a wide variety of sources, an essential aspect to help to address the needs/problems identified. Once the review had taken place, the justification for, or modification of, the initial plan of care could be highlighted. The final two activities in the section were a progress review with me as the link tutor, and a reflection on the process of learning so far, to be entered into a personal portfolio.

This common format was then continued through the next three sections, building on the initial plan of care. In section 2, 'Antenatal care through pregnancy', a review of test results was included to clarify normal biochemical ranges. As the exercise was simulated, a decision on when labour would begin and what type of labour/delivery was to be experienced was required to end section 2 and begin section 3, 'Care in labour'. In the spirit of midwives controlling their own learning experience, and in keeping with the PBL philosophy, this was left up to the individual studying each pack. Indeed, midwives were at all stages able to include scenario information that they wished to explore. A summary of labour needed to be devised before section 4 – 'Postnatal care' – was undertaken.

As time progressed a fifth section, 'Clinical practice links', was added to the pack. Although midwives were encouraged to review their work with peers as it progressed, this exercise remained a predominantly individual experience in terms of the learning achieved. Section 5 was designed to encourage a dissemination of personal learning to a wider audience. This involved an option to choose from either the production of a 'Guideline for Midwifery Practice', in which the underpinning for evidence-based practice existed, or another negotiated project if the midwife perceived this as being more valuable. Overall, it was felt that this sharing of knowledge could help to guide practice decisions in any new systems of care implemented.

With the package now almost complete, an introduction, a reminder of the 10 indicators of success, the overall aims and learning outcomes and a detailed guide on how to complete the work were included. Finally, a pre-pack use questionnaire and a post-pack completion questionnaire were devised in order to evaluate the success (or otherwise) of the project. In its final form, it was considered that this educational pack could indeed meet the following requirements:

- It was flexible enough to accommodate a multiplicity of learning needs and background experience, and mirrored the work patterns of a caseload-holding midwife.

- The self-directed nature of the study and the midwife being the one to direct events made the process manageable in practical terms.

- No *en masse* absence from the clinical area was necessary. In fact, it was while at work that much thought and discussion on possible care options and problem-solving strategies took place. Visits to other clinical areas were also made more frequently to collect and share information.

- After the initial production, the cost of each study pack was far less financially than that of attending study days or courses. It must be acknowledged though that while midwives used time in work to explore issues or problem-solve, they also undertook some work in their own time. This reflected a shifting of costs rather than their complete absence.

- The assessment and planning of care from the first antenatal visit to 28 days post-delivery could be carried out. The simulated nature of this exercise enabled the development of learning and practice strategies without the care of any woman being affected by the process.

- Personal learning needs could be identified and addressed in flexible and creative ways. Midwives were also in a position to develop their library skills.

- Reflection on learning was a process integral to each section.

- Hopefully a principle of 'lifelong learning' would be set as a result of this experience, achieving the project's goal.

Implementation

When the first draft of section 1 of the pack was complete in mid-1995, a request was made for midwives willing to try it out and give feedback on their experience. Twenty-two volunteers came forward to 'pilot' this section. As all midwives would be required to assess and plan care whatever scenario was chosen, many of the associated learning needs identified with this would automatically be addressed. The main priority was then to establish an area of practice in which each midwife initially wanted to develop his or her knowledge. Examples of some areas chosen included teenage pregnancy, drug use, antenatal screening issues, vegetarianism in pregnancy and preterm labour. A booking history scenario that would enable this focus to be taken was then provided. The process of feedback was mainly verbal, taking place in subsequent meetings. A number of issues were raised that helped to modify the way in which this and other sections of the pack were subsequently presented:

- One of the first general comments made was the need to be able to 'visualise' what a caseload-holding system would look like. Some items from the DoH (1993) report that covered this aspect were therefore included as pre-reading. A model of midwifery was also introduced as another way of dealing with this, and the common framework was found to be helpful.

- A common concern expressed was how information generated was to be recorded. In the case of the assessment and planning process, this was initially left open in the hope that user-friendly documentation might arise. Later, a general structure for data-recording was included in the study pack in the form of 'care plan' sheets for each section. For in-depth reviews and other activities, the production of a file of information was agreed as being the best way forward.

- The requirement for justification to be offered for care decisions was initially also found to be problematic. The midwives were trying to justify every single aspect of care, becoming bogged down in the process. It was agreed that general rationales would be offered for most things, to highlight the main purpose of an action. This would be supplemented by a more in-depth justification of one practice decision/action in each section. This successfully resolved this issue, making the whole process move forward more swiftly.

- The issue of how deeply to explore knowledge was also a significant factor. A balance was needed between the time it would take to investigate subjects in depth and the benefits of addressing a range of practice aspects. The midwives tended to accept that breadth rather than too much depth was most useful to begin with. However, this prompted the inclusion of an in-depth review of one subject area into the study process.

- Accessing the recommended readings was also time-consuming. As the opportunity to develop search skills was gained through undertaking the in-depth review, it was decided to hold the readings in a general file in the library.

- It was initially intended to add elements into the scenarios as the assessment and planning process progressed, but this was abandoned, for two reasons. First, it became too complicated and time-consuming to administer on an individual basis, and second, the midwives expressed a preference to make their own decision on how the scenario developed.

Having this type of feedback was invaluable in ironing out potential problems and the creation of a workable study pack. Another important element was the involvement of the librarian in the project implementation. She undertook to assist midwives in developing library skills and gaining confidence in using computer data sources such as CINAHL and later the Cochrane Database. Her help was integral to the success of the project, and midwife attendance at the library was noted to increase significantly. When the first two sections of the pack were complete in their modified form, a number of study sessions were held to introduce the rest of the midwives to the pack and its availability for use.

Assessment

When the packs were later used as part of formally conducted courses, a summative written assessment was introduced. Before this, formative 'self-assessment' was considered the best way to enable midwives to take responsibility for their own learning and instil self-confidence. The following strategies were part of this process:

- Self-assessment of learning was implemented, aided by the setting-up of group forums to discuss scenarios and plans, and verbally reflect on the learning process. Although it was originally intended to do this formally, it soon became apparent from the pilot review that the midwives were organising *ad hoc* groups for themselves, which changed spontaneously as different topic areas were covered. No attempt was made to interfere with this approach, and it was included as part of the process.

- Individual or group sessions with the link tutor also enabled learning and decisions made to be reviewed.

- If section 5 was completed, the production of an accepted evidence-based guideline for practice (or other project) would be a tangible way to demonstrate the achievement of learning outcomes.

The plan originally was to invite midwife managers, supervisors of midwives, GPs and other medical colleagues to submit their own plans/justifications for the antenatal first visit from the scenario details. These could then have been used by the midwives to compare the decisions made by themselves with those made by others. Although attempts to set up this mechanism were made, and initial enthusiasm was expressed, the plans failed to materialise. After a period of time, this part of the project was abandoned as unachievable.

Evaluation

While the 'pilot' run was evaluated verbally, it was necessary to devise a more formal method of evaluating the project overall. Pre- and post-pack use questionnaires were considered to be the most appropriate way of achieving this, eliciting both qualitative and quantitative data. Three main areas of evaluation were chosen, using a self-rating score for each. These were:

- The perceived level of confidence in ability to manage a personal caseload.
- The ability to access, review and apply knowledge.
- The extent of incorporating reflective accounts into the professional portfolio.

A 10 cm visual analogue scale enabled a rating score to be given.

For each element measured, a general hypothesis was formulated. In the case of one, it was that studying the caseload management pack will significantly increase the perceived level of confidence in ability to manage a personal caseload.

Similar hypotheses were formed for all the other elements evaluated. An initial analysis of data from 12 midwives completing the first two sections of the pack showed support for all the hypotheses in the direction predicted. Although the data produced were 'interval like', it was important to remember that they were still subjective ratings. A simple non-parametric test was used to compare differences in ratings between pre- and post-pack use. In the case of the hypothesis quoted here, the result was statistically significant ($T=1$, $P<0.001$ – one tailed). The qualitative data generated showed that the midwives felt it to be a useful, thought-provoking and relevant way in which to increase their knowledge and prepare for change. They did, however, find the workload relatively heavy, and there were some concerns expressed by those with little or no experience of self-directed learning. The involvement of the librarian was particularly useful here. She enjoyed being involved in the development process. The study pack was seen as providing just enough structure to give direction while retaining a significant amount of flexibility and challenge.

Progress

The hours available to work on this project were limited, it being a small part of a full-time workload covering both pre- and postregistration education. Hence it took around 18 months before all the pilot work was completed and the first two sections of the pack were finished. The remaining three sections were finally completed almost a year later. The aim had been to enable midwives to undertake a simulated process of assessing and planning care *before* changes to practice were introduced. As time progressed, it became evident that changes in practice reflecting the recommendations of the DoH (1993) report were not going to materialise. This arose from a combination of factors, but was sufficient to reduce significantly the motivation on the part of managers and midwives to continue with this form of study on a wide basis. The opportunity to put learning into practice was not going to become available, and this was a major stumbling block to the subsequent implementation of the project. It never really met its full potential in the way in which it was originally intended to. Even so, the work undertaken was not wasted. This study pack has been successfully utilised in a number of different ways. It is now a core unit within the BSc (Hons) Midwifery two-year part-time degree course at the University of Portsmouth. Students undertaking this course study the first two sections of the pack, focusing on antenatal care. The remaining sections are also being developed as individual study units that midwives are able to choose as options. It is being offered at the moment as a 1-week (equivalent) refresher course to meet the current statutory requirements for midwives continuing education (UKCC, 1998). It has also been incorporated into the Advanced Diploma 3-year preregistration midwifery course as a final year Level 3 unit. Its potential as a core component in a Return to Midwifery Practice course is also being considered.

Conclusion

This exercise was intended to be a direct simulation of caseload care-planning, and the evidence obtained suggested that it had the potential successfully to help midwives to prepare for this role. It could never have matched the process entirely, not least because it would always have lacked the individual and transactional nature of input that would have come from the woman and her family. Nor did it directly address the issue of developing the practical skills that would be necessary if caseload-holding were ever implemented. In addition, Andrews and Jones (1996, pp. 364) offer valuable comment when they state that:

> Students do not get to see the results of their problem-solving efforts... they can only assume the action taken was satisfactory or not.

This was particularly pertinent for this project. It was somewhat disappointing that the opportunity to see the effects of this learning in practice was never available. However, it was heartening to see those midwives who undertook parts of the study pack grow in confidence in terms of their perceived ability to carry out cross-continuum care, and of their development of a more self-directed learning approach. There was also a great deal of satisfaction in knowing that something useful could be developed from a close working relationship between clinical and education colleagues, a vital component of the effective development of midwifery practice, and of the effective development and implementation of PBL in the clinical area.

References

Andrews, M and Jones, P (1996) Problem-based Learning in an Undergraduate Nursing Programme: A Case Study, *Journal of Advanced Nursing*, **23**: 357–65.

Benner, P (1984) *From Novice to Expert: Excellence and Power in Clinical Nursing Practice*, Menlo Park, CA: Addison-Wesley.

Department of Health (1993) *Expert Maternity Group, Changing Childbirth* (Cumberlege report), London: HMSO.

Garbett, R (1996) Problem Power, *Nursing Times*, **92**: 1.

House of Commons Health Committee (1992) *Second Report on the Maternity Services*, Vol. 1 (Winterton Report), London: HMSO.

Rogers, J (1989) *Adult Learning* (3rd edn), Buckingham: Open University Press.

Stimson, L (1995) Caseload Midwifery – A Cost Benefit Analysis. *Modern Midwife* **5**(1): 12–14.

United Kingdom Central Council for Nurses, Midwifery and Health Visitors (1998) *Midwives Rules and Code of Practice*, London: UKCC.

Wise, J (1988) *Report on the Isle of Wight Maternity Services*, local publication for the Isle of Wight Health Authority.

Wise, J (1996) Preparation for Caseload Management, *Modern Midwife*, **6**(1): 15–17.

6

Group Dynamics and Disjunction in Problem-based Contexts

Maggi Savin-Baden

Introduction

One of the most important concerns when using PBL is the extent to which the groups in which students work and learn are effective. All too often, PBL is implemented within curricula with little real attention being paid to the relative costs and benefits of group-based learning. This chapter will argue that an understanding of group dynamics is vital not only for students involved in PBL, but also for the staff facilitating such groups. There is also little understanding of, or research into, the complex interplay of group and facilitator, and the way in which both change and adapt their roles and relationships as the PBL group matures. What will be presented first is an overview of the literature relating to the role of the facilitator and an exploration of whether the groups in which students learn are groups or in fact teams. The second part of the chapter will examine the notion of interactional stance and the concept of disjunction, exploring the impact of these issues upon group dynamics in problem-based contexts.

Facilitating PBL: what the literature tells us

There has been a considerable amount documented about the role of the facilitator in small groups (see, for example, Rogers, 1983; Heron, 1989; Eden and Radford, 1990; Jaques, 1991; Phillips and Phillips, 1993). Rogers (1983) suggested that the qualities of a good facilitator include realness and genuineness, accepting and prizing the learner and having the ability to offer empathic understanding. Jaques (1991) has argued that the role of the facilitator in learning groups is of one who has shared responsibility with the group for the learning, and that students and lecturer should accept one another for who they are rather than what they 'should' be. The bulk of the literature on the role of the facilitator in group-based learning therefore centres upon a personal relationship of respect and mutual trust between the learner and the facilitator. Yet there has been relatively little documented with regard to PBL.

In the field of PBL, Margetson (1993) has offered an in-depth consideration of the relationship between teaching and facilitation. He has argued that extreme interpretations of facilitation, which he has termed 'content free' (CF facilitation) cast the facilitator in the role of midwife. Such facilitators assist in the birth of the feelings and thoughts that students may have, and are prohibited from influencing the content of what is produced. Facilitation such as this is thus seen as a technical function that focuses purely on process and ignores content. Margetson has claimed that what is required is a notion of teaching and learning that is 'educative' and that avoids the extremes of content-only and process-only practice:

> Educative teaching *practises* a process-content whole which cannot be exclusively separated out into a component of process and a component of content. It is *facilitative* in encouraging the learner's active, co-operative participation in extending, enriching, and transforming what is most valuable in existing meaningfulness – that is, it facilitates the learner's extension of his or her own understanding and knowledge *in relation* to the knowledge and understanding of others both current and past. (Margetson, 1993, pp. 168)

Despite this sound argument, Margetson has not explored the complexities of diverse facilitator roles and styles within groups at differing stages of group development. Facilitator roles and styles may affect the kind of educative teaching on offer. A further issue when considering group change and development, and the role of the facilitator within that, is the notion of learning context. It is often assumed that a learning context is something that can be defined according to the situation and perhaps even the disciplinary area of study. Yet learning contexts are transient in nature, and much of the real learning that takes place for students occurs beyond the parameters of presented material. Since educational programmes are temporary environments, it is important to raise students' awareness of the changing nature of the learning environment, peers and lecturers, and themselves within it. Therefore, a recognition of the relationship between staff's espoused theories and theories-in-use, in conjunction with students' perceptions of the formal learning context, is key to facilitating students' ability to manage group learning effectively.

In spite of such helpful and challenging perspectives in this field, there has been relatively little *research* into the role and effectiveness of PBL facilitators. Those studies undertaken fall into two areas: staff perceptions of PBL and staff effectiveness in PBL programmes. The issues raised within the context of these two areas exemplify the increasing interest and concern about staff involved in PBL programmes and the lecturer's ability to facilitate groups effectively.

Staff perceptions of PBL were explored in a study undertaken by Neame (1982), who examined the academic roles and satisfaction in a problem-based medical curriculum. He identified three areas that were seen to contribute to staff satisfaction. These were the acceptance of the educational philosophy of PBL, the way in which PBL was implemented and the outcomes of using PBL. Neame found that staff were committed to the philosophy and satisfied with the implementation, and that a beneficial outcome of PBL was seen to be interdisciplinary collaboration. An important issue identified by Neame was that staff involved in the programme over a greater period of time were more committed to PBL than were those who had been involved for a shorter time. It would thus seem that familiarity with PBL as a way of teaching may be an important factor in staff satisfaction and effectiveness in PBL programmes.

Gijselaers and Schmidt (1990) found that lecturer functioning had a direct causal influence on small group tutorials, which in turn influenced students' interest in the subject matter. However, Dolmans *et al.* (1994a) developed an instrument to assess lecturer performance in PBL tutorial groups. The lecturer evaluation questionnaire comprised 13 statements reflecting the tutor's behaviour. Although this instrument was found to be valid and reliable, it did not account for changes in group process or for the need for different types of facilitation at different stages in the course. A further shortcoming of this study was the lack of definition of what counted as an effective facilitator role. A more recent study carried out in the same department (Dolmans *et al.*, 1994b) argued that lecturer evaluation should be embedded in a broader faculty development programme. This should include the development of the formal role of the facilitator, the stimulation of faculty dialogue, the design of a lecturer reward system and learning opportunities for the staff. The authors concluded that the study demonstrated that putting effort into a faculty development programme resulted in increasing attention being paid to teaching activities within the curriculum, a finding supported by a recent study in the UK (Murray and Savin-Baden, 2000).

It is clear from these studies that the role, satisfaction, effectiveness and training of staff in PBL programmes is still an under-researched area that requires a detailed consideration of the differing types of lecturers' roles at different stages in the group process, and an exploration of differing tutor roles across disciplines. Studies need to be undertaken into how tutors manage their evolving role within groups, and into the way in which they are prepared for involvement on PBL courses.

Groups or teams?

Throughout the literature on PBL, little has been discussed about whether students are working in groups or teams. Learning groups gained popularity in higher education in the 1960s and have continued to gain ground since. However, the move towards a market model of higher education has paralleled the increasing demand for accountability to the public and state, and for greater vocational relevance. Closer links between higher education and industry have promoted changes in curricula generally and supported an emphasis on the development of personal qualities for life and work. Employers are thus demanding graduates who are not only competent to practise, but also bring with them computer skills, an ability to think critically and the aptitude to work in teams (cf. Chapter 1). If we then explore the difference between learning groups and working in teams, it will be possible to see whether it is in fact groups or teams that are required to equip students effectively for the world of work.

Teams are often equated with games, such as football and basketball, in which the members have different roles but equal status. For many years, the word 'team' has also been used in commerce and industry to denote a group of people engaged in a specific task with a clear remit, but who make decisions together. Yet in higher and professional education, this term appears to be used little, the more loosely bounded expression of 'group' being preferred. The problem here is that to talk of PBL groups implies that a cluster of people have come together with a collective perception, with shared aims and having made the choice to work and learn together. This is often not the case since students have been allocated to groups, and the task is invariably predetermined. In addition, some students only undertake PBL because it is a condition of their choice of course or subject. Groups are often places where joining is part of the process of becoming cohesive, where there is a sense that people choose to be present and that they have an option to leave at any time.

Teams differ in that they demand a different kind of ethos, culture and commitment. To belong to a team usually means that there is a common purpose and a limited membership, and that the team has the power to make decisions. Teams have a focus, a set of team rules, and are time limited. Thus, a team is organised to meet together; it has a context and a task. As such, it would seem that the term 'team' is more appropriate to what occurs in most PBL seminars because there is a focus and a remit, and because much of the learning that occurs evolves through the ways in which the team make decisions about what and how they learn. However, before exploring issues connected with the working of the team, it is important to explore what individuals bring to the team and the ways in which their roles, behaviours and perspectives on team learning can impact upon the team as a whole.

Interactional stance

There is often a sense that the role that staff and students adopt when involved in team-work differs from other roles at university and in the practice setting. Such roles, and the behaviours that are often assigned to them, have been described in detail by authors such as Belbin (1993). While Belbin's role profiles are useful for designing and managing teams whose purpose and identity is defined by a task focus, such a model does not capture the complex interplay of factors occurring for students in the kinds of learning team that are in operation in problem-based contexts. What is needed instead is a set of concepts that together encapsulate the richness and ambiguity of problem-based team learning and interaction. Research into PBL demonstrated that staff and students' ability to work and learn effectively within teams was affected by the position they chose to take up within PBL team – their interactional stance (Savin-Baden, 1996).

Interactional stance depicts the way in which a learner interacts with others within a learning situation. It refers to the relationships between students within teams, and staff–student relationships at both an individual and a team level. An interactional stance encompasses the way in which students interpret the way in which they as individuals, and others with whom they learn, construct meaning in relation to one another. The way in which one student may theorise about another student within a team setting reflects his interactional stance, as does the way in which a student acts and speaks in interacting with other students. Interactional stance is also a notion that encompasses the means by which students engage with, and attribute meaning to, the processes that occur in teams. It is subsequently through reflection upon these processes that students make sense of their own learning.

Interactional stance: a case example

Nursing students at one UK university found that working and learning in PBL teams had helped them to see the value of shared learning and the advantages of solving problems and difficulties together. In particular, students valued the opportunity that PBL offered them both to discuss with their peers problems that had emerged from practice, and also to learn to work collaboratively, which had not been an opportunity on offer in other areas of the nursing curriculum.

Emily was a student who had found learning on her own in other areas of the curriculum a difficult task. She had spent the first year of the course writing up lecture notes and revising for examinations. Although she had passed the course thus far, she believed she had forgotten most of what she had learned, and only had six ring binders full of notes to show for her first year of being a nurse. Although when she went on practice placements, she felt that she had the basic skills needed for her stage of training, she constantly felt ill equipped to transfer the knowledge from examinations and essays to the work place. In her second year, Emily began PBL and discovered that learning to solve and manage problems with and through others in the team helped her to retain the information more effectively than before, and to use other people's experience to understand concepts and practice when she encountered barriers to learning.

Such support, which developed throughout teams across the cohort, meant that students were able to spend time reflecting upon their placements and working through difficulties together. By obtaining a number of differing perspectives on how to address a problem, students were enabled to return to their placement with a number of new strategies and a greater understanding of their experiences. Thus, issues that may initially have appeared complex and unresolvable for an individual became a group project through which group members facilitated each other in making sense of individual concerns.

The impact of interactional stances on teams

Within the overarching concept of interactional stance, there are four domains, students tending to adopt one of these in the context of the team in which they are learning. Thus, the relationships between students within teams, and staff–student relationships at both an individual and a team level, are affected by the different domains that individuals adopt. Yet students do not just adopt one domain at all times. The way in which students operate in teams is affected by a number of factors. For example, students' perspectives about what counts as knowledge, their view of themselves as learners and what they believe they do or do not bring to the team, their prior experience of learning in teams and their concept of the role of the facilitator will all affect the domain that they adopt. The four domains of inter-actional stance are presented in Figure 6.1.

Individualism	Validating personal knowledge	Connecting personal experience through interaction	Transactional dialogue

Figure 6.1   Domains within interactional stance

These four domains can be delineated as follows.

Individualism

'Individualism' depicts the notion that some students see learning within the team as an activity that is valuable only in terms of what they as an individual can gain from it. These students place little value upon collective learning experiences and are more concerned that they may forego marks by expending effort on sharing tasks and information within the group rather than by working alone. Interactional stance as captured within this domain is characterised by the individual placing himself at the centre of the value system. Thus, learning within the team is an activity that is valuable only in terms of personal gain for the individual.

Phil was a student who had fixed ideas about the method by which the problem should be solved, and the way in which he wanted the feedback report (which was to be assessed) to be produced. Phil found it difficult to accept that other people in his group also had their own ideas and that his idea was not always the best one. He felt disadvantaged by not being in control of the work and invariably offered to be the group member who collated the report so that he could ensure that the group's chances of obtaining the highest marks were maximised. Phil thus used strategies ensuring that he as an individual would gain the best possible marks, even if this meant overruling group opinions and collective values.

Validating personal knowledge

Much of the real learning that occurs through PBL happens through team interaction, but this is not often rewarded in academic terms. The domain of validating personal knowledge captures the idea that through the experience of being heard within a team, and being valued by other team members, individual students learn to value their own knowledge and experience. Students tend to speak of 'making sense', 'connecting' and 'seeing things in a new way', all within the context of the team. Thus, for many students the team learning process has more meaning than learning that is formally assessed.

Rachel, for example, discovered that in one problem scenario, she was one of the experts in her team in paediatrics because of her prior experience of working in this field. Being an expert helped her to develop confidence and realise the value of her prior experiences, both to herself and to the team.

Connecting personal experience through interaction

Students in this domain tend to speak of the way in which learning and reflection within teams enables them to make sense of their own experience as learners. Thus, students use teams to make sense of the interrelationship of their problem-solving processes, their prior experience and the new material being learned.

For example, Bill's prior experience of didactic methods meant that he could not understand how he could learn through discussing the problem, or how students' differing approaches to problem-solving could possibly produce a cohesive group and an effective answer. Personal reflection, along with reflection and discussion with others, enabled Bill to explore not only the unresolved set problem, but also his difficulty of being at an impasse in the problem-solving process. Through dialogue with his peers, he was able to consider how to tackle the given problem and thus integrate that which had been incomprehensible and unfamiliar into his life-world.

Transactional dialogue

In this domain, the team serves as an interactive function for the individual. Here, dialogue is central to progress in people's lives, since through it values are deconstructed and reconstructed, and experiences relived and explored, in order to make sense of roles and relationships.

For example, Douglas was a student for whom learning to work in a team was about learning not only how to learn in a team environment, but also about democracy, loyalty and effective team-work. He learned that his focus had to be the achievement of the task with a spirit of co-operation, rather than putting his needs before the achievement of the task. Although, in terms of the course, he realised that the aim was to solve the given problem, he saw learning in teams in the broader context of offering the opportunity to understand and explore other people's perspectives. Douglas talked about this in terms of 'learning to exist with people' and 'choosing to get on with them'. For him, learning with and through others was something that required effort and had to be worked at, and it was only through this that he could hope to understand other people's perspectives. Dialogue offered Douglas the opportunity to explore differing ways of knowing that would ultimately offer him a deeper understanding of the way in which roles and relationships affected his effectiveness as a future professional.

Thus, interactional stance encompasses students' interpretation of the way in which they as individuals, and others with whom they learn, construct meaning in relation to one another.

Yet the domain that students occupy can reflect not just their own perspectives and motivation, but also their view about how effective their team is, its purpose and the extent to which the team and the facilitator prompt and enhance effective team learning. In order for teams to work effectively, it is important that they are clear not only about their individual role and perspectives in the team, but also about the aims and goals of the team as a whole. It is only through such understanding that effective team motivation and commitment can be achieved.

Managing PBL teams

Anyone who has been part of a team knows just how hard it can be to get all the members dedicated and motivated. Achieving team motivation demands commitment, and what underpins this is that the whole team must believe in the value of both the team-work itself and the task being undertaken. PBL can be implemented for a whole host of reasons (see, for example, Savin-Baden, 2000), and opportunities for team-building are invariably the first things to be erased from a curriculum if there is a perception that there is inadequate time for content delivery. This is often the first step towards a breakdown of the team. Teams need to be built, they need secure foundations, and at the outset they need to be clear about their own aims and goals in relation to the overarching curriculum expectations. Simultaneously, individual members of the team need to be clear about their own roles: why they are there and what is expected of them. Building teams will, in the first instance, help the team to develop a sense of commitment that will sustain it through demanding periods of growth and development. Yet in our fragmented and incoherent society, there are difficulties with notions of commitment and team-work. The shifts towards self-directed learning, autonomous learning and students as 'consumers' tend to promote a notion of individualism that signals an end to dialogue and, with it, a devaluing of collaborative and dialogic approaches to learning. This is reinforced by governments and health services who concentrate on meeting targets, which often bring with them a focus on outputs rather than outcomes, and the task rather than the process. Yet both an elected government and a collection of ward staff need to learn to work together as an effective team.

Teams are motivated when they can see a value, purpose and sense of reality in the task. Therefore, task and process in PBL teams need to be inextricably linked to real-world situations, which will secure students' inquisitiveness and offer them feedback on their overall effectiveness. Nevertheless, it is often the case in health sciences curricula that students are expected to learn about ' the normal person' before they are permitted to explore disease and illness. The irony is that the motivation of most students on such courses is to learn about illness – that is what they feel they are there for. Students can learn about what counts as normal in the process of exploring illness. Doing this will engage students' motivations, which will in turn enhance team commitment. Teams are also motivated by feedback and reward, yet few problem-based seminars are rewarded in real terms. Students need to see assessment as part of the learning process as well as part of their development towards being effective health professionals who can work in teams. However, in order to ensure team commitment, students need to work together through a team-building activity to develop ground rules to which they all feel able to be bound and committed. Figure 6.2 illustrates the ground rules that emerged from one collaborative team exercise.

The facilitator and the team

In the context of moving towards PBL, many staff become confused about what it means to be a lecturer and/or facilitator in higher education. This may at first seem to be related specifically to the shift in role from lecturer to facilitator in the context of PBL, yet it would seem that it is much more complex than this as staff are expected to manage increasingly diverse and ambiguous roles. For many staff engaged in PBL, the transitions from lecturer to facilitator demand revising their assumptions about what it means to be a teacher in higher education. This is a challenge to many as it invariably demands the recognition of a loss of power and control when moving towards being a facilitator, since:

the facilitator is one who assists in the student's learning, even to the extent of providing or creating the environment in which that learning may occur, but he (she) is never one who dictates the outcome of the experience. (Jarvis, 1995, p. 113)

- The team will be committed to its membership in ways that will encourage the sharing of information and a realistic self-appraisal of the team and the individuals within it.
- The team will create a safe and supportive learning context that promotes trust and commitment within the team.
- Team members will give and receive feedback towards one another that is supportive and constructively critical.
- Confidentiality of issues shared and discussed within the PBL team will be maintained within the bounds of the team itself.
- There will be a commitment to punctuality as defined by the team.
- The team will develop its own commitment to attendance and decide upon the ways in which it will manage the non-attendance of its members.
- The team will utilise self-regulation mechanisms and means of ensuring that equity is maintained across the team in terms of status, workload and contribution to the team.
- Respect for contributions made by other members, both verbally and in writing, will be maintained as far as possible.
- Team members will produce agreed work (as decided by the team) on time.
- The team should seek to clarify, and contribute to, the definition of the role of the facilitator in the team.
- The team should take shared responsibility for the progress of the process and outcomes of the team.
- Team members should be willing to learn from other members of their team.

Figure 6.2   Example of a team's ground rules

It is becoming increasingly apparent that staff seem to receive little support or guidance in ways of managing transitions in the change process. Yet many staff have suggested that the cycle shown in Figure 6.3 is the type of cycle through which they move as they facilitate PBL teams.

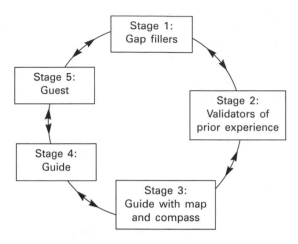

Figure 6.3   Shifting roles for staff

Staff's perspectives on their transitions can be described as follows:

- *Gap fillers:* Staff believed that they were there to help to alert students to gaps in the subject content being researched and/or to offer mini-lectures in the seminars to help to fill those gaps.

- *Validators of prior experience:* From being gap-fillers, staff believed they moved to a role of helping students to bring their prior experience to the team in order to utilise and value such experience.

- *Guide with a map and compass:* Staff felt that, in this stage, they were using their own perspectives to guide students through the problem scenario because they had the 'right' knowledge to guide students to the 'right' places to acquire and learn the knowledge and skills required.

- *Guide:* The next transition for staff was that of being a guide helping students to consider information and skills but not always directing their tack; instead, staff's role was that of a co-ordinator of knowledge and skill acquisition across the boundaries of both.

- *Guest:* Staff described this stage as being an orchestrator of opportunities for students, their role being a somewhat privileged one as they facilitated students in a learning debate around the problem scenario, and in their quest for skills and abilities.

It is pertinent to note that staff roles shifted according to the group process, and that there were times when staff cited examples of moving back into the roles of gap-filler and validator of the students' experience (Savin-Baden, 1998a). Furthermore, many of them found self-management to be a complex task while they were simultaneously helping students to manage their own transitions towards learning approaches that few had previously encountered. However, the relational aspect of learning has been valued by many students (Savin-Baden, 1996). They have argued that getting to know a facilitator through learning in problem-based teams, and experiencing a form of learning that appears to be more informal than the lecture-based components of the curriculum, has enhanced their learning experience. For such students, informality has brought with it a sense that staff and students have shared aims in learning. Students have asserted that this enabled them to feel that the learning was collaborative, not just in terms of collaboration within the cohort, but also between staff and students. Yet despite this, there are a number of issues of which facilitators should be aware when working with and managing PBL teams:

- Acknowledge the shift in roles and relationships for staff and students engaged in student-centred learning.
- Recognise that facilitator–student expectations of one another will be in a process of change and mutual simultaneous shaping.
- Be aware that teams are often less stable and predictable than the literature on team theory implies.
- Regularly ensure that both the facilitator and the team are clear about, and revisit and possibly revise, the ground rules.
- Appreciate that it is important for both lecturer and students to value students' prior experiences.
- Ensure that the team keeps an accurate record of each individual's allocated task to ensure accountability and commitment to the team.

- Develop strategies in advance for managing high-level conflict within the PBL team that cannot be managed by the team itself.
- Realise that facilitators need to be critically self-aware of their role within the team and in the interventions they make.

Faultlines in teams

Faultlines are the places where fissures appear in structures and institutions, systems and communications, because of weaknesses. We can all point to faultlines: places where things persistently go wrong. Breakdowns commonly occur as a result of the same catalyst and with characteristics similar to those seen on the previous occasion. Over time, these can result in increasingly haphazard decision-making and inaccurate assumptions about what is required within the team. Faultlines in PBL teams tend to occur in three key but interrelated areas: learning, communication and evaluation. It is, however, the learning faultline that we will explore here.

The learning faultline: disjunction

Disjunction can be defined as becoming completely 'stuck' in learning, as feeling fragmented. The result is frustration, confusion and often a demand for the 'right' answers. Disjunction is not something that can be seen as a single incident of anger or confusion; instead, it is multifaceted in nature and 'emerges out of mutually interacting influences' (Weil, 1989, p. 112). Disjunction occurs when there is a conflict between an individual's biography and his or her current experience. Thus, prior (learning) experiences no longer enable people to make sense of their current situation, and they become consciously aware that they do not know how to act, which prompts a search for new meaning and understanding.

Four key ways of managing disjunction in teams

Students deal with disjunction in a number of different ways, which means that the conflict, ambiguity and incoherence experienced by individual students cannot be defined by distinctive characteristics; there are, however, some general trends. What seems to be apparent is that disjunction is dealt with by students, in one of four ways, through forms of decision-making that are conscious and/or unconscious. Thus, students may opt to retreat from disjunction, to temporise and thus choose not to make a decision about how to manage it, to find some means of avoiding it and thus create greater disjunction in the long term, or to engage with it and move to a sense of integration.

Retreat

Students may choose not to engage with the process of managing disjunction. They want to avoid engaging with the struggles connected with disjunction and often retreat behind some form of excuse that means that they do not engage with the personal or organisational catalyst of the disjunction.

Temporising

Students who do not directly retreat from disjunction may adopt an indecisive or time-serving policy. They acknowledge the existence of disjunction and also that they have to engage with it in order to enable an effective transition to take place, but they decide that it is preferable to postpone making any decision about how to manage it.

Avoidance

In this situation, students do not just temporise, but adopt mechanisms that will enable them to find some way of circumventing the disjunction. The result will be that although the student has found a means of bypassing the disjunction, this may have taken more effort than engaging with it.

Engagement

Engaging with disjunction requires that students acknowledge its existence and also attempt to deconstruct the causes of disjunction by examining the relationship with both their internal and external worlds. Through this reflexive examination process, students can engage with what has given rise to the disjunction, and they can then shift towards a greater sense of integration.

Guidance for managing disjunction for students and teachers

Students have to learn to manage disjunction themselves, but if they fail to manage it successfully, it is likely that the issue(s) that was the initial catalyst for the disjunction will continue to become progressively disabling and inhibit further progress until it is managed effectively. (Particular catalysts to disjunction are discussed elsewhere, for example Savin-Baden, 1998b). Figure 6.4 offers some techniques to help staff and students faced with disjunction.

- Discuss the existence and nature of the disjunction with students and staff. The understanding of what is taking place often helps students in particular to manage the disjunction more effectively than if they had not been aware of the characteristics of disjunction.
- Explain that disjunction is a common occurrence for students on problem-based programmes.
- Offer support that enables a shift away from disjunction, through listening, providing support and expressing positive expectations
- Encourage the PBL group to examine prior instances of disjunction and explore what previously helped and hindered the shift away from disjunction.
- Explore their prior experience of learning, which may allow students to reframe their disjunction.
- Investigate the extent to which disjunction has been prompted by the difference between what has been espoused and what happens in practice.
- Offer opportunities for reflection upon learning and practice.
- Acknowledge that the burden for managing disjunction is not wholly the responsibility of the students, and ensure that there are mechanisms in place to support this.
- Remember that peer relationships and/or practical guidance from within the problem-based group can provide support and can become the means by which individual students are enabled to manage their disjunction.

Figure 6.4   Tips for managing disjunction

It is important that disjunction is managed effectively. Mechanisms should be in place so that disjunction *can* be managed, and in ways in which it *is* or *becomes* enabling, so that the burden of responsibility for managing that disjunction is not left wholly with the students.

Summary

This chapter has explored the importance of acknowledging that students in PBL work in teams rather than groups, places where there are clear aims and goals, and where individuals are clear about their role and purpose within the team. The concept of interactional stance demonstrates that, in the process of building teams, it is important to understand the domains that students adopt within the team. Such an understanding will help staff and students to develop a sound comprehension of team roles and relationships, which will in turn prompt the effective management of individual and team disjunction. For educators using PBL, the effective management of disjunction will mean not just that students will develop generally applicable competences, but that they will also be able to adapt them and critique their value throughout their professional lives. It will mean that change is seen as a feature of their professional lives rather than a fault, and that critique becomes the touchstone of professional self-management. These issues of team dynamics, interactional stance and disjunction are central concerns to those adopting and enacting PBL in curricula.

References

Belbin, R M (1993) *Team Roles at Work*, Oxford: Butterworth-Heinemann.
Dolmans, D H J M, Wolfhagen, I H A P and Snellen-Balendong, H A M (1994a) Improving the Effectiveness of Tutors in Problem-based Learning, *Medical Teacher*, 16(4): 369–77.
Dolmans, D H J M, Wolfhagen, I H A P, Schmidt, H G and Van der Vleuten, C P M (1994b) A Rating Scale for Tutor Evaluation in a Problem-based Curriculum: Validity and Reliability, *Medical Education*, 28(6): 550–8.

Eden, C and Radford, J (1990) *Tackling Strategic Problems: The Role of Group Decision Support*, London: Sage.

Gijselaers, W H and Schmidt, H G (1990) Development and Evaluation of a Causal Model of Problem-based Learning. In Nooman, A M, Schmidt, H G and Ezzat, E (eds), *Innovation in Medical Education, An Evaluation of its Present Status*, New York: Springer.

Heron, J (1989) *The Facilitator's Handbook*, London: Kogan Page.

Jaques, D (1991) *Learning in Groups*, London: Croom Helm.

Jarvis, P (1995) *Adult Learning in the Social Context* (2nd edn), London: Croom Helm.

Margetson, D (1993) Education, Pedagogy and Problem-based Learning. In Viskovic, A R (ed.), *Research and Development in Higher Education 14*, Sydney: Higher Education Research and Development Society of Australasia.

Murray, I and Savin-Baden, M (2000) Staff Development in Problem-based Learning, *Teaching in Higher Education*, **5**(1).

Neame, R L B (1982) Academic Roles and Satisfaction in a Problem-based Medical Curriculum, *Studies in Higher Education*, **7**(2): 141–51.

Phillips, L D and Phillips, M C (1993) Facilitated Work Groups: Theory and Practice, *Journal of Operational Research Society*, **44**(6): 533–49.

Rogers, C (1983) *Freedom to Learn for the 80's*, Columbus, OH: Charles C Merrill.

Savin-Baden, M (1996) Problem-based Learning: A Catalyst for Enabling and Disabling Disjunction Prompting Transitions in Learner Stances?, Unpublished PhD Thesis, University of London Institute of Education.

Savin-Baden, M (1998a) Fugitives or Nomads? The Changing Roles and Relationships of Staff and Students in the Context of Global Study, Paper presented at Tomorrow's World: The Globalisation of Higher Education, Society for Research into Higher Education Annual Conference, University of Lancaster, 15–17 December.

Savin-Baden, M (1998b) Problem-based Learning, Part 3: Making Sense of and Managing Disjunction, *British Journal of Occupational Therapy*, **61**(1): 13–16.

Savin-Baden, M (2000) *Problem-based Learning in Higher Education: Untold Stories*, Buckingham: SRHE/Open University Press.

Weil, S (1989) Access: Towards Education or Miseducation? Adults Imagine the Future. In Fulton, O (ed.), *Access and Institutional Change*, Buckingham: SRHE/Open University Press.

7

Introducing Problem-based Learning into Distance Learning

Bob Price

Introduction

Pausing to consider what problem-based and distance learning have in common, it is tempting to argue that both play a role in liberating the learner. While PBL empowers the student to discover information for her- or himself, and to value that which is on offer through experience, distance learning makes education possible, even if a teacher is not close to hand (Rowntree, 1986). Both problem-based and distance learning claim to be student centred and facilitate the student in becoming a critical and independent thinker (Barrows and Tamblyn, 1980; Evans and Nation, 1989). Beyond this, however, there are significant difficulties in bringing the two educational approaches together. That which is assumed to be pivotal within PBL (for example, a facilitative tutor who has sustained and non-directive contact with students; Little and Ryan, 1988; Creedy and Hand, 1994) is not usually practical within distance learning. Distance learning, with its emphasis upon delivering a multitude of information in an accessible manner, seems the antithesis of learning by discovery. In short, PBL would seem to emphasise education as a process, while distance learning, by choice or necessity, is often portrayed as a product-driven system of learning.

This chapter will explore the extent to which distance learning and PBL may work together to enrich the education of nurses and midwives. With imagination, and some forethought, distance learning systems (material and student support) can be designed to help students to develop useful PBL skills. To do this, however, it will be necessary to question the tenets of distance learning within the UK. These have stemmed from the considerable success of the British Open University since the early 1970s, and are centred upon delivering high-quality information (facts plus examples of cognitive debate) through text-based materials. Within the classic open university model, student participation within the materials has often been confined to periodic activities directed by text, while tutors have been assigned roles relating to the interpretation of theory in practice and promoting student networking (Murphy, 1995; Price, 1997). What has been fundamentally flawed within the classic model of distance learning is an unclear, often inadequate utilisation of the tutor-counsellor, and a belief that learning materials, however well written, should be directed towards teaching, rather than the facilitation of learning.

To clarify this exploration of the possible benefits of combining problem-based and distance learning, we shall illustrate the debate using a project undertaken within the BSc in Nursing Studies by distance learning at the Royal College of Nursing Institute. This degree serves the needs of registered nurses who wish to top up to a first degree and whose work or personal needs dictate that distance learning is the preferred means of study. The programme is modular, each module being supported by a regional tutor-counsellor and assessed by a piece of course work. Students study this programme across the UK and overseas, and are offered the option of joining regular Saturday group tutorials. Those students who cannot attend the tutorials maintain contact with their tutor using a variety of means, including fax, email, letter and telephone. In excess of 300 students have studied on this programme.

Theorising in practice

At the end of the first year of studies, students complete a module called Exploring the Art and Science of Nursing II. This module has been conceived of as a nursing scholarship module that focuses upon practice knowledge and the ways in which theory, philosophy and research may be combined to make a difference to practice. The module offers three projects focusing upon PBL, concept development and theory critique respectively. Students choose a project to major in, while being required to read material associated with the remaining projects. The PBL project is called Theorising in Practice (Price, 1998) and is designed, through the facilitation of the tutor-counsellor, to help students identify, analyse and then explore tentative solutions to a clinical challenge that they are encountering. Theorising in Practice (Price, 1998) has been expressly written to help students value their practice knowledge, and to challenge the romantic curriculum that has developed within nursing (Bradshaw, 1998). By the end of the 15-week module, students prepare a detailed problem analysis, which includes a consideration of the options for future nursing action.

Unlike classical PBL, which typically begins at the start of an education programme, preceding formal teaching about component subjects (Barrows, 1985, 1996), Theorising in Practice (Price, 1998) is embedded within an established and theory-driven curriculum. Students have been taught the tenets of nursing philosophy, current nursing theories and nursing research as it is conducted within a variety of traditions. Unlike classical PBL, which extends over many months or even years of study, this project is time limited to 15 weeks. The project was conceived as helping students to develop complementary skills within nursing, and its scope as limited, respecting the fact that this was (to our knowledge) the first attempt to deliver PBL opportunities through distance learning within British nursing. While we were excited by the possibilities of an inductively led education, we were not convinced that the approach was as yet well developed enough to risk a whole distance learning curriculum within it (see Biley and Smith, 1998, for a review of a more ambitious project). We have been mindful that Exploring the Art and Science of Nursing II was a 'designated module' that students had to pass. It followed that students should be offered the elective of a PBL project, and many of them (69 out of a cohort of 101 students) accepted it.

Writing PBL materials

A number of things characterise the classical approach to distance learning materials (Figure 7.1). While they are written in an accessible manner (for example, addressing the reader as 'you') and designed to minimise confusion (they have a low 'fog factor'), it is nevertheless assumed that they must teach the student a subject. Distance learning material writers face a dilemma as they must second-guess the background, needs and experiences of their readership, who may come from a wide variety of nursing fields (Clarke and James, 1994). Because of this, classical distance learning materials tend to be conceptual or thematic, explaining theory that could ostensibly be applied to a variety of situations (for example, leadership, consultancy, research and models of nursing). The writer uses illustrations (from his or her own practice), activities (which encourage the student to explore the chosen concept locally) and off-prints (articles that expand upon the concept or debate it in some way) in order to help students to gain a command of the subject matter. Distance learning is therefore quintessentially about comprehension, synthesis and application. At its best, it may help the student to transfer key concepts to new areas of practice.

Planning to write PBL materials is itself therefore inherently problematic. If the writer chooses to write about concepts (a content of what *should* be learned), he has failed at the first hurdle. The material simply replicates the problems that were criticised by Barrows and Tamblyn (1980), in which students are told the theory and invited to make practice fit with that theory. The material then remains inherently deductive, with a priori theory applied to a variety of situations, fitting more, or often less, well. What then should be written about PBL, as a process rather than a product, within the materials of a distance learning module? How can materials be devised that help students to gain some shape or purpose for their own discovery, without unduly inhibiting the process of learning? Furthermore, how can materials be written that leave an appropriately imaginative role for module tutor-counsellors, who remain important facilitators of learning (Morgan and Morris, 1994; Price, 1997)?

- Written in an open style, addressing the reader directly.
- Written with due concern for accessibility (often a low 'fog factor').
- Incorporating activities that it is assumed that the student pauses to complete.
- Incorporates written feedback after the activity, second-guessing what the student may have discovered and offering an author's experience or view.
- Written in conceptual terms (explaining and debating concepts that could apply to a wide variety of nursing contexts). The readership may come from varied backgrounds.
- Presented with clear structure (the material detailing the aims/learning outcomes and signalling the layout of the material that will follow).
- Periodically refers students to additional, often contrasting references (frequently supplied as off-prints).

Figure 7.1   Characteristics of classical distance learning material

Theorising in Practice (Price, 1998) was written to provide students with the tools with which to conduct their own problem analysis. The material, of necessity, provides a framework for thinking about problems, but one which is also open to adjustment and development by the student him- or herself. First, students were encouraged to explore the different types of knowledge, often tacit, that they might use in practice decisions (Eraut, 1990) (Figure 7.2). It was not assumed that all of Eraut's (1990) types of knowledge would be used in any one problem, or that each type of knowledge would have equal meaning for the student. Nevertheless, the notion of marshalling what the student already knew, about the situation, the players and the processes, that typically occurred in relation to the problem seemed to be an important part of the problem analysis process.

We purposively avoided the use of Carper's (1978) ways of knowing within this project. Whatever Carper may have intended for her work, it has subsequently achieved icon status within the romantic nursing curriculum and is often used to suggest how nurses should think about problems, as well as the range of practice issues with which they may concern themselves. Theorising in Practice (Price, 1998) was designed to minimise the ideological

---

Knowledge of people
While this can seem imprecise, nurses anticipate how others may feel and react based upon their experience of how others have reacted before. A knowledge of people may be culturally informed; that is, some reactions and values are culturally determined and therefore easier to anticipate

Knowledge of processes
This is the knowledge of how things get done (for example, making a referral to a specialist practitioner or liaising with social services to organise longer-term rehabilitation)

Empirical knowledge
Abstract knowledge that can be used to inform professional values, patient or client education and prioritisation of care. For example, a knowledge of how diabetes mellitus affects the human body, and therefore the client's lifestyle, is empirical knowledge. A knowledge of drugs and their impact upon the body, and of the theory of grief reactions, is also empirical knowledge

Control knowledge
This refers to the ethical and professional handling of emotions. Control knowledge is knowledge not about how to manipulate others, but about how to handle one's own emotions within stressful settings. Control knowledge is therefore based upon understanding oneself, one's beliefs and values, and those issues or stances that are likely to seem personally uncomfortable

---

Figure 7.2   Types of tacit knowledge that may underpin practice
(after Eraut 1990)

steerage of students' learning, so that after their prior education, they could formulate their own valuation of theory and philosophy. To this end, types of knowledge (Eraut, 1990) and other component tools were selected in part because nurse education had not treated them as icons of what should be.

The second component of written material concerned itself with the process of decision-making in practice. Not only did decision-making play a key role in problem analysis and the identification of solutions, but it could also lie at the heart of the problem in the first place. We sought to make students aware that decision-making was not necessarily a rational or evaluated process, and that a problem analysis might usefully incorporate a careful review of how decisions had been made. To this end, students were given an account of how practitioners form hypotheses about what they see in clinical practice, and how such working hypotheses are then tested out as new information comes to light, or the practitioner makes specific enquiries (Elstein and Bordage, 1988). Students were encouraged through activities to explore their own decision-making steps, as well as sensitively to question the basis of how decisions were made and what the impact of decisions might mean for others. Underpinning this material was the belief that experienced practitioners could (and should) articulate their practice decisions, particularly within an evidence-based practice world in which professional status might be open to scrutiny by others (Bradshaw, 1998). While intuition was accepted to be a part of many clinical decisions, it was not accepted that it should preclude an analysis of practice. On the contrary, intuition was argued to be at best a partial defence when practitioners were invited to justify practice within a court of law or similar setting (Price, 1999).

The third component of material read by students concerned itself with the frames of reference that nurses might use to approach and investigate a problem. We were keen to help students to understand that the perception of a problem could be affected by a number of filters (assumptions and preconceptions), which served to set parameters on the size and nature of the problem, or indeed to determine whether it was seen as problematic at all. To illustrate this, we drew students' attention to the ways in which nurses often created and used a perceptual set when coming on shift (Parker and Wiltshire, 1995). Students were encouraged to set down clearly, therefore, the beliefs, values and goals that affected their approach to clients and situations, and to discuss these with colleagues (both nursing and from other professions) in order to discover the differing perceptions that could shape the problem in hand.

Finally, we paused to consider the ways in which different nursing philosophies, theories or research might be incorporated either into the analysis of the problem or as a possible contribution towards a solution. For example, Conway (1996) has highlighted the different world-views that nurses operate with, and argues that this significantly affects how nursing expertise is defined. Such philosophical underpinnings could both significantly affect the ways in which a problem was defined, and inform the suggested solutions to that problem. A nurse operating within the humanistic existentialist world-view might be expected to take a very different view of a problem to a nurse who saw it in terms of specialist nursing knowledge. Within the material, we examined ways of thinking about the utility of nursing philosophy, theory and research. It was accepted that research did not invariably offer truth, and that philosophy could also limit opportunities for problem-solving. Formal nursing theories (of whatever level) might help nurses to conceptualise what they were doing, but they could equally hinder practical solutions.

As with other distance learning materials, Theorising in Practice (Price, 1998) was read by a wide range of critical readers prior to being issued to students. It was immediately acknowledged that the material was very different, and that it might come as a shock to students who had been used to a more 'fact-giving' approach to education. Tutor-counsellors, however, did not see this as a problem. On the contrary, it quickly became apparent that this material was seen as relevant to practice, and that it would fuel conversations between students and tutors. Whereas in other modules, tutors had explained that they found their role ambiguous, within this module, they identified a number of key roles associated with the PBL project.

Providing support

Tutor-counsellors supporting students on the Exploring the Art and Science of Nursing II module had been used to fulfilling four key roles:

- Helping students to interpret their module reading within a local context.
- Role-modelling the critical reading of materials.
- Helping students to plan the demonstration of their learning through course work assignments.
- Assisting students to cope with the pressures of work and part-time study.

Because of the PBL project, however, they received additional briefing on their role as a facilitator of learning. Specifically, it was explained that they should adopt a supportive, but non-directive, stance as students identified problems that interested them, and then began the journey (with materials) through the problem analysis process (Barrows and Tamblyn, 1980; Doring *et al.*, 1995). Tutor-counsellors were encouraged to help students to identify for themselves new sources of information and additional skills in data-gathering and analysis. They were asked to emphasise the importance of sharing their ongoing analysis with colleagues at work and through the tutorial group. Where students were unable to attend tutorials, such networking of ideas was managed at a distance. For example, two students in Thailand and one in Canada formed a problem-solving group, analysing problems through the medium of email.

To the above extent, the facilitative approach to PBL appeared to mirror much of the work that tutor-counsellors had always done with distance learning students. While they might operate in a slightly less directive manner, they nonetheless sought to help students to make sense of their own situation. There were, however, a number of fundamental and only partially foreseen consequences of asking tutors to support students through a PBL process within distance learning education.

The first (and pleasant) surprise was associated with the way in which other practitioners within the students' practice setting became involved in the problem analysis. Theorising in Practice (Price, 1998) was read not only by the student, but in some instances by up to a dozen other practitioners: nurses, physiotherapists, doctors and related healthcare practitioners. They reported to the tutor-counsellor that the student's studies were manifestly practical and might be of benefit to them too. For this reason, tutor-counsellors found themselves being approached as problem analysis facilitators not only for the student, but also for a number of his or her associates. This surprised tutor-counsellors, who felt both flattered by the requests from problem-solving groups, yet unsure of their expertise in group facilitation. Tutor-counsellors observed that while in many groups there was clear evidence of progress through problem analysis, and the creation of one or two early solutions, there was also a wish that the tutor would continue to facilitate the group after the module had concluded.

Even in situations where students later reported that they did not feel that they had substantially solved the clinical problem, they did attest to the supportive, sometimes cathartic, benefits of working in a multidisciplinary group to address a problem. As one student observed:

> We had a patient who mobilised unexpectedly and often unsafely because he was confused and disorientated in hospital. Until this project we had simply restrained the patient and felt that we had failed. The project prompted us to think again about why he was suddenly getting up and wandering, so that we started to learn the signs that said Ted needs a walk. No... we didn't completely solve the problem, but we did feel good about ourselves, not having to restrain Ted to quite the same extent. (Gregg, student)

Tutor-counsellors and we ourselves had underestimated the sense of relief that a PBL approach might offer to practitioners. Education delivered through such a framework was seen as tangible and 'real world', and, contrary to what might have been expected, was not evaluated solely in terms of whether the problem was resolved.

The second (and rather more problematic) sequela of introducing the new approach into this module of learning was that students engaged in problem-solving study started to dominate the attentions of the tutor-counsellor. Other students (completing concept analyses or a critique of nursing diagnoses) found that discussion at tutorial became dominated by discussion of problem analysis in progress. They reported that these students were clearly 'heavily engaged' in their studies, but that the enthusiasm could carry the attentions of the tutor-counsellor along. It rapidly became apparent that there was a need for tutor-counsellors equitably to ration their formal tutorial time. This was achieved in a number of ways, but often meant that informal problem-solving groups continued after the tutorial had completed.

If the students experienced enthusiasm for their own PBL, they also experienced periodic anxiety. In particular, this was associated with the first stages of problem identification, and then occurred again at the end, when the students came to write up their analysis. There was no shortage of problems that the students felt that they could analyse, but tutor-counsellors quickly became aware that there was a need to contain the problem chosen to what might be manageable within the module time-frame. Problem containment, while not a feature within classical PBL curricula, was a key concern within this case study.

Problem containment was achieved in a variety of ways, but this usually included helping the students to see their problem as a stage or aspect of a larger problem. Students were encouraged to select relatively discrete problems, not because we anticipated that they should necessarily have resolved the problem by the end of the module, but because we felt the need to help them to manage a modest palette of ideas and possibilities when they were inductively learning so quickly. We were aware that the classic pattern of group discussion, and then independent enquiry, before returning for further cycles of discussion (Rangachari, 1996), was not readily arranged within distance learning, and that problem containment at the outset was critical if students were to feel a sense of progress.

The challenge of writing up a problem-based analysis was made less daunting by examples of problem analysis (at different stages of refinement) being offered within Theorising in Practice (Price, 1998). Nevertheless, even though sample problem analysis reports were offered, students found it initially unsatisfying to write up an analysis that did not necessarily have a problem resolution at the end. Such pieces of academic writing could feel 'unfinished', and indeed many students went on to offer a problem solution some months after the module had ended.

To encourage students with their assignment work, tutor-counsellors illustrated the criteria that would be used to assess their work. We had already sanctioned the showing of marking guidelines within tutorials, emphasising that assessment was in this instance not based on whether the problem had been resolved but on whether the student had demonstrated insight into the PBL approach. Students were assured that personal insights, dispassionately written, would be an important part of the assignment. Some tutor-counsellors encouraged students to write short paragraphs of problem analysis, and evaluated these with the student before final submission of work. At the close of the module, such measures appear to have been effective, because the distribution curve of grades favoured B (60–69 per cent) with 10 students out of 69 achieving an A grade (over 70 per cent) and only two students failing the assignment.

The 'so-what?' of problem-based distance learning

While the above account of PBL within a distance learning programme suggests that this approach is both possible and indeed desirable, a number of points deserve careful attention. In particular, questions need to be asked about the fit of PBL as an educational approach within the broader nurse education curriculum. We need to consider whether PBL should be the sole philosophy underpinning a curriculum or whether it in fact represents a complementary approach to more traditional, perhaps deductive, learning within nurse education. These are not idle points of debate, as has been made clear by the publication of a consultation paper on the integration of theory in nursing practice by the Chief Nurse (England) (NHS Executive, 1998), and by some of the more recent debate on the cost-effectiveness of higher education-based nurse education.

In addition to the philosophical questions, we need to consider what this case study teaches us about the preparation of materials and support services within distance learning. Just as distance learning has served to highlight some of the opportunities and limitations associated with PBL, so PBL has enabled us to question the treasured assumptions about how distance learning does or should work. The experience has been symbiotic.

The philosophical question goes right the way back to the critique of medical education in North America during the 1960s and 70s (Barrows, 1996). To what extent does the traditional curriculum, with its teaching of theory and then the application of theory to practice, remain appropriate to the needs of practitioners? If it is proven to be wanting, is this necessarily also true of the postregistration curriculum? Nurses who are already qualified practitioners, and who later extend their education further, arguably already have considerable knowledge of the 'how to' of problem-solving. Perhaps these nurses' needs are different because they seek a judicious mix of new knowledge (with which to feel authoritative) and new skills (through which they may react to or lead practice development within the future) (Brookfield, 1987; Jones and Brown, 1991).

Our perspective has been eclectic. We believe that educational approaches should remain tools to an end, and that the student's success in learning is of greater importance than arguments about which approach *should* dominate the curriculum. There seems to be some merit in assisting students to learn both inductively and deductively, because this in fact mimics the world of nursing and practice development. We are not yet convinced that to have learned nursing through a theory-led curriculum precludes students from also learning other aspects of that curriculum through a PBL, inductively led approach. The students involved in this case study appear to have made a successful, if at times anxious, transition between the different approaches to learning. The learners have been reflexive enough to understand why the experience of learning was different, and why such learning was important to their education as a whole. Despite the argument made by Barrows (1996) and others, it has been apparent that these nurses were able to set aside their past education, and to question again the ways in which theory, philosophy and research may have influenced their perceptions of problems and the problem-solving process.

Indeed, we would wish to argue that PBL, at least within distance learning programmes, may benefit from being introduced not at the beginning of the curriculum, but after the student has been equipped with a variety of concepts that may or may not seem relevant to the problem in hand. Students who have exercised their understanding of abstract concepts may be better equipped to manipulate these and concepts derived from their experience, within a problem analysis and solution sequence. Learners starting from such a position certainly seem less likely to be anxious about their knowledge base, and quicker to explore afresh the assumptions that have shaped nursing practice in the past (Spouse, 1998).

Having observed this, however, we also argue that there is a case for a greater use of PBL within the distance learning (and quite possibly the campus-based) curriculum. At present, distance learning nursing curricula have tended to emphasise a theory-driven approach, and there has been scant opportunity for nurses to explore practice knowledge. While a great deal is argued about the merits of reflective practice, and reflective practice education, with or without clinical supervision (see, for example, Manley and McCormack, 1998), it is by no means clear that such education actually assists nurses to change practice. On the contrary, many nurses simply appear to add a new layer of theory to their studies, about what reflection is or should be, and what counts as an appropriately scholarly reflection.

This poses the question of which subject fields or areas of nursing practice are especially amenable to PBL. Within the distance learning nursing curriculum, can adjustments be made that permit students to develop their powers of inductive and deductive reasoning side by side? Certainly subjects such as research and education in practice appear to be well suited to PBL approaches. For example, while research has traditionally been taught as a subject to be appreciated (that is, analysed and understood), it has rarely been presented as a curricular subject that is to be used. Nurse academics have misgivings about how research (particularly of post-positivist, naturalistic design) can be utilised in practice. Allusion is made to the fact that qualitative data research may 'illuminate' practice (Koch, 1995). Curriculum planners have tended to shy away from exploring techniques by which nurses may not only critique research, but also form judgements about the utility of research within a given context. PBL seems well suited to this aspect of research education. Indeed, PBL may become central in making evidence-based practice a reality, illustrating how research is selected for use within problem analysis and solution formation.

A similar case can be argued for education in practice, that pertaining to the education of both colleagues and clients. It is arguable that the current approach (that is, here are theories of learning, teaching and assessment; go and apply them in the clinical area) is particularly unhelpful. Clients cannot be assessed like student nurses, and little consideration is given to the impact that stress, information overload and sensory deprivation may have upon the client or student's learning environment (Lanoe and Price, 1997). There is considerable opportunity here for distance learning education on this topic to start from the experiential end of the spectrum and to examine what learning is like within a given environment, before tailor-made teaching and assessment strategies are then devised.

Learning subjects such as evidence-based practice and education in practice, through distance learning and a PBL approach, is, however, a qualitatively different experience. The graduates of such a programme may be multiskilled, and perhaps more confident about changing practice in the future, but they will have been challenged to learn in a much more active way than is currently the case within distance learning. Precisely because such learners are required to bring practice into academic discussion and assessment work, they are also required to engage in more philosophical debates. When the module assignment is about their problem, and their journey towards resolving that problem, they cannot (with success) think or write superficially. There is scant opportunity for the student to skip the activity set within the distance learning text, because that activity may in fact be integral to understanding their own problem. Failing to engage in the activities is not an option when the non-completion of such activities may profoundly affect the students' ability to address the situation that they confront.

PBL is inherently challenging, because it engages both the student's mind and his or her emotions. Students savour the success of making progress and sense the frustration of meeting a blind alley. There are close parallels to be drawn with research work leading to a dissertation. Students cannot be sure, at the outset of their work, what the outcome of their endeavours will be. They must shape the learning that follows and cannot expect the teacher to shape it for them. Even for the inquisitive and academically able student, this is a taxing as well as a worthwhile way to learn. It may suit some students' learning styles better than others, and because nursing needs practitioners with a variety of skills, and many different ways of learning, we are wise to be cautious about the level and speed with which we introduce PBL.

So how much PBL should we introduce? At this stage, I believe that there is a case for introducing an increasing proportion of PBL the further into the course a student progresses. Within the first year of the BSc in Nursing Studies, the ratio of two theory-driven to one practice-driven module seems correct. Within the second year of studies, however, the ratio could usefully be reversed. A case can be made for offering two modules that are practice focused, and inductively led, with one final module (the dissertation) that retains a more traditional and deductive stamp (this currently being a research literature review). Balancing the volume of problem-based and traditional education is based upon assessing students' readiness to accommodate different ways of learning, as well as new subjects of scholarship. We wish to argue that PBL requires a maturity on the part of the student that may not yet be apparent within preregistration early-stage programmes, and that is equally in short supply as students tackle a new programme of learning within a different mode of study.

Rethinking distance learning

Irrespective of whether PBL becomes a prominent feature within distance learning nurse education curricula, its lessons should be understood with regard to the writing of distance learning materials and the organisation of tutor-counsellor support. If distance learning education is to operate at levels above comprehension, we are forced to find ways of prompting students to do more than just read their text. It is naïve to imagine that students will complete the activities set for them to do, if (a) the text proceeds to offer an author's solution, and (b) superficial learning is reinforced by an assessment system that fails to connect in a coherent way with text activities and tutor-counsellor-linked discussions. The current classical approach, writing material that is conceptual and explanatory, is an inadequate solution to the problems of learning that nurses face. We need to write material that helps them to think for themselves, neither suggesting what they *should* think nor leaving them to wonder what counts as legitimate learning. What has been discovered in Theorising in Practice (Price, 1998) is that it is possible to write substantial material that helps students to discover their own knowledge. It is also possible to write material that helps students to connect such practice knowledge with that which is taught more formally in other modules.

Similar lessons pertain to the role of the tutor-counsellor. Just as student learning from the text page has often been passive and superficial, so the learning potential associated with tutor-counsellors has also been left underexploited. It is insufficient to suggest that the tutor-counsellors help to interpret material and then address the expressed needs of the student group. Within this framework, the expressed needs of the students may move towards the superficial. Instead of addressing the real problem of understanding the material being studied, and what that can mean for practice, the student considers how an account (dressed for examiner consumption) can be prepared as an assignment. The student learns not how to learn, but how to present an argument that he or she may not have fully considered. In such circumstances, distance learning, as other modes of study, then fails the purpose of nurse education – to facilitate learning among practitioners who will need to learn to grow and develop as professionals.

PBL provided tutor-counsellors within this case study with a glimpse of a more creative and constructive relationship with students. The tutor was encouraged to become a process consultant, assisting the students to engage in issues that they knew more about – their practice. The expertise of the tutor-counsellors was not spuriously claimed to be about the problem subject (be that insulin injections or promoting continence), but was instead embedded in their training in reasoning and learning. Tutor-counsellors reported that there was a clearer focus for their work, and that students engaged in learning as well as asking about assignment presentation. While the concern to pass an assignment understandably remained, assignment answers seemed to stem from a deeper level of insight into practice.

Conclusion

There is a tradition that conclusions in academic papers, be they chapters in books or papers in journals, are about disclaimers and reservations. The author is concerned to sound cautious, and appropriately dubious about what his or her discoveries might mean for the profession more widely. Well, this chapter has its disclaimers too, and its cautionary notes. The exploration into whether PBL can be utilised within distance learning nurse education has involved a calculated risk that students might struggle to learn in this way, but in the end it has also been a surprisingly successful one. We have been relieved that students and tutors have benefited. We believe that the case study has taught us almost as much about distance learning as it has about PBL. Certainly, we have begun to understand the limitations of classical distance learning education, as presented during the past three decades within Britain.

We have been heartened, especially by the prospect of arranging education in the future that develops nurses' ability to reason deductively and inductively in concert. We are unwilling to drop the benefits of traditional education, or to abandon the gains offered by PBL, as illustrated in this case study. We think that nurses have the capacity, with support and at the right stage in their education, to benefit from a mix of educational approaches. The learner who understands how he or she learns, as well as what is worth learning, is a powerful practitioner who can continue to learn long after the programme of education has finished. Central to this process within distance learning is the artful writing of new materials and the development of tutor-counsellor roles. We have learnt that PBL can help us to celebrate teaching – the facilitation of learning by experienced and committed nurse teachers who know that their work is central to the success of the student.

Nurse education now faces many of the criticisms that faced medicine several decades before. We have the opportunity to counter the criticisms of nurse education if we are prepared to address the integration of theory in practice and to help nurses explicitly to reason about their practice. PBL became a part solution within medicine. There are a number of faculties that have founded their education programmes upon it. Significantly, however, there are more medical faculties that have rejected PBL as the solution to integrating theory and practice. Perhaps with the benefit of such hindsight, and understanding our profession's propensity to turn tools into ideologies, we may yet gain the benefits of PBL without turning it into something that it need not be. Certainly, within distance learning, there is a place, a pivotal place, for PBL within our programme and that of many others.

References

Barrows, H (1985) *How To Design a Problem-based Learning Curriculum for the Pre-clinical Years*, New York: Springer.

Barrows, H (1996) Problem-based Learning in Medicine and Beyond: A Brief Overview, *New Directions for Teaching and Learning*, **68**: 3–12.

Barrows, H and Tamblyn, R (1980) *Problem-based Learning: An Approach to Medical Education*, New York: Springer.

Biley, F and Smith, K (1998) 'The Buck Stops Here': Accepting Responsibility for Learning and Actions after Graduation from a Problem-based Learning Nursing Education Curriculum, *Journal of Advanced Nursing*, **27**(5): 1021–9.

Bradshaw, A. (1998) Defining 'Competency' in Nursing, Part II: An Analytic Review, *Journal of Clinical Nursing*, **7**(2): 103–11.

Brookfield, S (1987) *Developing Critical Thinkers: Challenging Adults To Explore Alternative Ways of Thinking and Acting*, Milton Keynes: Open University Press.

Carper, B (1978) Fundamental Patterns of Knowing in Nursing, *Advances in Nursing Science*, **1**(1): 13–23.

Clarke, B and James, C (1994) The Evaluation of Flexible Modes of Learning in Nurse Education and Practice, Conference Paper, Nurse Education Tomorrow Conference, September, University of Durham.

Conway, J (1996) *Nursing Expertise and Advanced Practice*, Dinton: Quay Books.

Creedy, D and Hand, B (1994) The Implementation of Problem-based Learning: Changing Pedagogy In Nurse Education, *Journal of Advanced Nursing* **20**(4): 696–702.

Doring, A, Bramwell-Vial, A and Bingham, B (1995) Staff Comfort/Discomfort with Problem-based Learning: A Preliminary Study, *Nurse Education Today* **15**(3): 263–6.

Elstein, A and Bordage, G (1988) Psychology of Clinical Reasoning. In Dowie, J and Elstein, A (eds), *Professional Judgement: A Reader in Clinical Decision Making*, Cambridge: Cambridge University Press.

Eraut, M (1990) Identifying the Knowledge which Underpins Performance. In Black, H (ed.) *Knowledge and Competencies: Current Issues in Training and Education*, London: Scottish Council for Research in Education, and Alison Wolffe, University of London.

Evans, T and Nation, D (1989) *Critical Reflections on Distance Education*, London: Falmar Press.

Jones, S and Brown, L (1991) Critical Thinking: Impact on Nursing Education, *Journal of Advanced Nursing*, **16**(5): 529–33.

Koch, T (1995) Interpretative Approaches in Nursing Research: The Influence of Husserl and Heidegger, *Journal of Advanced Nursing*, **21**(5): 827–36.

Lanoe, N and Price, B (1997) *Education Applied to Practice: A Study Guide*. London: RCN Institute.

Little, P and Ryan, G (1988) Educational Change through Problem-based Learning, *Australian Journal of Advanced Nursing*, **5**(4): 31–7.

Manley, K and McCormack, B (1998) *Exploring Expert Practice: A Study Guide*. London: The RCN Institute.

Morgan, C and Morris, G (1994) The Student View of Tutorial Support: Report of a Survey of Open University Education Students, *Open Learning*, **9**(1): 22–33.

Murphy, M (1995) Open Learning: The Manager's and Educationalist Perspective, *Journal of Advanced Nursing*, **21**(5): 1016–23.

National Health Service Executive (1998) *Integrating Theory and Practice in Nursing*, Report Commissioned by the Chief Nursing Officer/Director of Nursing, London: DoH.

Parker, J and Wiltshire, J (1995) The Handover: Three Modes of Nursing Practice Knowledge. In Gray, G and Pratt, R (eds), *Scholarship in the Discipline of Nursing*, Melbourne: Churchill Livingstone, pp. 151–68.

Price, B (1997) Defining Quality Student Feedback in Distance Learning, *Journal of Advanced Nursing*, **26**(1): 154–60.

Price, B (1998) Theorising in Practice, Part 1 of Bellman, L. and Price, B (eds), *Exploring the Art and Science of Nursing II: A Study Guide*, London: RCN Institute.

Price, B (1999) *Updating the Theory–practice Debate: An Occasional Paper*. London: RCN Institute (Clarifying Theory for Practice – distance learning module).

Rangachari, P (1996) Twenty-up: Problem-based Learning with a Large Group. *New Directions for Teaching and Learning*, **68**: 63–71.

Rowntree, D (1986) *Teaching through Self Instruction: How To Develop Open Learning Materials*, London: Kogan Page.

Spouse, J (1998) Scaffolding Student Learning in Clinical Practice, *Nurse Education Today*, **18**(4): 259–66.

8

Assessment and Evaluation in Problem-based Learning

Di Marks-Maran and B. Gail Thomas

Introduction

This chapter will explore two issues that are fundamental to PBL programmes: assessing and evaluating PBL. Because the terms 'assessment' and 'evaluation' mean different things to different people, we will begin by offering our definitions of these two educational terms. When we speak of assessment, we are referring to knowing that our students have learned. Assessment measures the learning impact on the individual student. Evaluation, on the other hand, is about the overall quality and value of the programme from the perspective of all the stakeholders. The two concepts are inextricably linked but will be examined separately in this chapter.

Assessment in PBL

In all educational endeavours, one of the important considerations is congruence between the values and practices underpinning the different parts of a curriculum. For example, there should be congruence between the overall philosophy or intention of the programme and the nature of the approaches to learning that are taken in the programme. Additionally, there needs to be congruence between the approach to learning and the approaches to assessment used to measure the achievement of learning. Nowhere is this more true than in PBL. The literature offers a number of reasons why PBL is seen, by some, to be the approach of choice. Engel (1991, p. 23) suggests that:

> While higher education has a long tradition of fostering scholarship and of valuing knowledge for its own sake, the primary responsibility... is to assist students in their development of the capability to benefit from and cope with modern life, and to contribute productively to their society.

Margetson (1991) suggests that, in subject-based learning, expertise is defined in terms of subject content; that is, to be an expert is to know a lot of content. In PBL, however, expertise is measured by the ability to make sound judgements about what the problem is in a professional situation, how to prioritise problems and how to solve (or prevent) problems using evidence.

In summary, there appears from the literature to be a number of identified intentions or purposes of PBL. These are:

- Learning is structured through the integration of subjects within the discipline being studied.
- Learning is structured around real-life problems, scenarios or situations that students would be expected to be able to solve or manage in the real world of work.
- PBL deliberately sets out to help students to develop open-mindedness, to be reflective and critical, and to learn actively.
- PBL enables practitioners to become evidence based.
- Students develop the ability to synthesise, analyse and evaluate.
- Students become independent learners who can direct their own learning.
- PBL fosters group co-operation in the learning process.

If these are the key intentions or purposes of PBL, they raise challenges for the course designer and the problem-based tutor with regard to the assessment of learning. As suggested by Margetson (1991), in subject-based learning, expertise is determined through content and then the assessment of learning is based on measuring the extent to which content has been learned. Given the list of purposes or intentions of PBL, it is clear that merely testing content knowledge is not enough to assess the wide range of cognitive and transferable skills inherent in PBL. A congruent assessment strategy in a PBL curriculum needs also to test some or all of the other intentions or purposes identified earlier.

A problem-based assessment scheme must therefore be designed to measure the following aspects of student performance:

- Course content, or storehouse of knowledge.
- The ability to demonstrate the use of appropriate knowledge to solve or prevent real-life problems or situations (to prioritise problems).
- A reflective self-assessment ability.
- The ability to question and demonstrate open-mindedness.
- The ability to provide evidence justifying decisions that have been made.
- The ability to analyse a situation critically, synthesising from a wide range of sources and evaluating the decisions made.
- The ability to work independently yet in co-operation with a group.

The test of the success of learning through PBL lies in assessing all (or as many as possible) of these purposes of PBL.

The literature related to assessment in PBL

When the University of Newcastle Medical School in Australia first began delivering its medical education programme through PBL, they adopted an assessment tool called the Medical Independent Learning Exercise (MILE). This method of assessment was specifically designed rigorously to assess students' content learning as well as their competence with regard to independent learning (Feletti *et al.*, 1983). Assessment using this tool was based on either real or simulated patient problems and gave students the opportunity to seek, use and discriminate between resource materials appropriate to the management of the patient problem. The tool was tested for statistical reliability and validity, showing high internal consistency. Feletti *et al.* (1983) concluded from their study of the MILE assessment tool that its main strength lay in its ability to measure accurately the relative success of the learning *strategies* adopted by the student as well as to assess the knowledge (content) gained.

Hodgkin and Knox (1975) first devised the modified essay question (MEQ) on behalf of the Royal College of General Practitioners. Feletti (1980) described the MEQ as an assessment method in PBL and explored reliability and validity issues surrounding it. Knox (1980) suggests that the MEQ is a technique that can measure abilities and attitudes that other techniques cannot. Very simply, the MEQ is an account of an evolving event as a case study. The case study is narrated as it occurs (Knox, 1980), and points are selected at suitable times and places within the case study at which questions are asked. The students are required to provide decisions that are justified from evidence. Knox describes the technique as a useful learning approach within the curriculum, as well as an assessment tool. When used for assessment purposes, students' responses to questions during the scenario are measured against the responses that a panel of experts in the field perceive to be the most appropriate responses. Knox suggests that MEQs can be merely factual, which defeats their purpose: assessments requiring only factual responses can be elicited through a number of other assessment methods. The MEQ, on the other hand, opens up possibilities for exercising 'intelligent guessing' (Knox, 1980) and other abilities that more realistically reflect the realities of clinical work. Thus, a successful MEQ can and should contain a mixture of questions, all related to the scenario, that provide a balance between factual, diagnostic, decision-making and evaluative questions.

Silén (1998) describes the MEQ examination process used at Linköping University in Sweden. It is based on the assumption that the assessment process must match with the concept of learning and knowledge within the theoretical framework of PBL. Their MEQ-style examinations attempt to use the problem-solving process as the basis for assessing understanding as an outcome of learning. The PBL examination aims to reveal the student's level of understanding related to qualitative differences in managing the situation and the enquiry, reasoning and critical thinking processes. At Linköping, assessment is seen as a vehicle for learning within a problem-based curriculum.

Norman (1991) makes the point that one of the central roles of PBL is the nurturing of problem-solving skills. He suggests that assessment methods need to be devised that explicitly measure these skills. Norman describes the MEQ as an assessment method that addresses process knowledge of the 'What would you do next?' form.

The Triple Jump is an assessment technique for testing a range of PBL intentions: problem-solving ability, content knowledge, the synthesis and application of knowledge to new clinical situations, the justification of decisions and evidence-based practice. As such, it is widely used as an assessment tool in PBL programmes (Painvin *et al.*, 1979).

The Triple Jump is a problem-based, oral assessment method. Used extensively in some medical schools, the Triple Jump involves an individual student being given a case scenario or patient problem with a certain amount of information relating to the patient. The student reads the situation/problem and verbally presents his or her first impressions and deductions from the information given to the tutor. The student then identifies some critical issues that he or she wishes to follow up in order to make a diagnosis, identify treatment or solve a problem. The tutor engages in a dialogue with the student to help him or her to tease these out, asking probing, challenging open-ended questions. This is step 1 of the Triple Jump process. Step 2 involves a period of independent study by the student during which the student uses the resources available to explore the identified issues or problems that were identified in step 1. The student then returns to the tutor to verbally present the newly formed evaluation of the situation, including deductions, analyses and identification of the interactions. Step 3 involves the justification of decisions, with reference to the evidence. When step 3 is over, the tutor gives feedback to the student directly, offering praise and constructive criticism where necessary and appropriate (Pallie and Carr, 1987). In some institutions, the student's own tutor conducts the Triple Jump, while in others, it is undertaken by an independent tutor.

Norman (1989) states that many of these PBL assessment methods have not been tested for content validity. For him, the most important question is whether it is possible to assess problem-solving skills independently of the knowledge component of the programme. Norman (1991) undertook a quasi-experimental study that found that the MEQ assessed nothing different from a parallel multiple choice test. From this work and other literature, it appears that PBL is not about the development of problem-solving skills independently of knowledge. Instead, PBL concerns knowledge that is acquired in the context in which it will be used in the future. However, PBL is to do not with assessing students' knowledge of facts in isolation (a feature of traditional subject-based programmes), but with the assimilation of new knowledge into existing structures. Norman and Schmidt (1992) referred to studies in cognitive psychology and suggested that the ability to learn is influenced by many factors. They concluded that one of the strongest of these factors is the similarity between the context in which the knowledge was first learned and the context at the time the learned knowledge is subsequently retrieved. What Norman (1991) seems to be saying is that, in successful PBL, course designers and tutors need to make a serious and conscious attempt to match these two contexts.

Some hybrid PBL programmes use the problem-based tutorial process but retain tradition examinations as the vehicle for assessment. Martensen *et al.* (1985) demonstrated that where this is the case, when biochemistry knowledge was tested through a short-answer question examination, both PBL and subject-based students showed no difference in their results in these short-answer tests at the end of the programme. However, when the tests were repeated 2–4 years later, those who had undertaken a PBL course had a significantly higher degree of retention (60 per cent higher) of the biochemistry knowledge than did those who had learned biochemistry in a subject-based curriculum. This would suggest that it is the PBL process itself that is significant to long-term learning and retrieval, rather than the assessment methods used. Finally, Norman (1991) cautions that, although at the very minimum students in PBL must demonstrate that they do as well as non-problem-based students, it is expected that PBL provides something extra – added value – to this. The assessment of knowledge is not enough, the other intentions of PBL (identified at the beginning of this chapter) needing to be assessed as well.

Swanson *et al.* (1991) take this a step further and argue the need for 'process-oriented assessment methods'. They suggest that communication, problem-solving skills, the acceptance of responsibility for learning, learning to learn and the selection and use of appropriate resources for learning are the key features or purposes of PBL. Therefore, these need to be assessed alongside the acquisition of knowledge. Swanson *et al.* (1991) offer a number of such process-oriented assessment methods, critically evaluating each. One such approach is the use of tutor, peer and self-rating scales. Although this method is used widely in PBL, studies into the validity of tutor, peer and self-assessment have indicated that validity is poor (Boud, 1988; Rezler, 1989). These studies seem to indicate that overall impressions can be made through peer, tutor and self-assessment but that differentiation between distinct skills is unlikely.

Swanson *et al.* (1991) also examined what they refer to as 'unobtrusive measures' of assessment. This involved quantifying the number of library books and journals that were borrowed, analysing computer records to see how many literature searches were undertaken, and asking students to keep learning logs to capture and summarise their learning activities. They suggested, however, that these unobtrusive measures were more likely to be useful as curriculum evaluation tools rather than individual student assessment tools. Swanson *et al.* conclude that the Triple Jump is probably the most reliable and valid process-oriented tool. However, psychometric and validity tests carried out on the Triple Jump suggest that it is probable that students' perfor-mances vary extensively from problem to problem because of the content-specificity (Painvin *et al.*, 1979; Powles *et al.*, 1981; Swanson, 1987; Swanson *et al.*, 1987). This means that many Triple Jump assessments across a wide range of content areas would need to be undertaken to provide a valid assessment of learning.

Because many of the process-oriented assessment methods are psychometrically suspect and largely untested for validity, process-oriented methods should be supplemented by outcome-oriented approaches such as the modified essay, well-constructed, reli-able multiple choice tests, short-answer tests and invigilated exam-inations. One problem that has been encountered in some attempts to implement PBL is that university validation systems are unfamiliar with some of the more process-oriented assess-ment methods, as well as that staff are sometimes uncomfort-able allowing programmes to deviate from the standard assessment methods associated with traditional subject-based learning programmes. This accounts for the wide number of programmes in which the delivery method used is PBL but the assessment methods rely on subject-based methods. Assessment methods that are being designed as part of problem-based programmes must prove to be valid and reliable but, according to much of the literature, this is not the case.

A case study in the assessment of a PBL programme

In 1998, The Wolfson Institute of Health Sciences at Thames Valley University developed a preregistration BSc (Hons) in Nursing course. An intensive staff development programme was provided for those members of the academic staff who would be developing and delivering the programme. Part of this development programme explored the nature of assessment in PBL.

In discussion with the two PBL consultants employed to work with the team, four principles were agreed as the basis for developing the assessment strategy:

● The need for a rich and stimulating mixture of assessment methods across all modules of the programme.
● The belief that assessment should be a vehicle for learning and not just an 'add-on' at the end of the module.
● The need for the assessment methods to be congruent with, and reflect, the PBL approach and the purpose of PBL.
● The need to ensure that all assessments demonstrated that the students had achieved the module learning outcomes.

Three modes of assessment were selected that reflected the above principles as well as some of the intentions of PBL outlined earlier in this chapter. The three modes of assessment selected were: a problem-based/problem-solving case study; a modified essay and a theory–practice portfolio of evidence. Since there are three modules per academic year within the programme, the team decided to use one of these in each of the modules within each year. The exception to this was the modified essay, which appears only in one module in year 1 and one module in year 2. Each of these assessments increases in size and complexity from year 1 to year 3. The final module, at the end of year 3, is assessed using a dissertation project. In addition to these theoretical assessments, a clinical practice profile of skills is completed for all modules. The exception is in those modules which use the theory–practice portfolio, in which case the portfolio incorporates both theoretical as well as clinical assessment.

Table 8.1 gives a summary of the assessments for this PBL programme.

The theory–practice portfolio

The theory–practice portfolio is a collection of evidence provided by the student over the length of the module. The nature of evidence presented is made clear to the students, and criteria for evidence are derived from the module learning outcomes and the purposes/intentions of PBL. The criteria for evidence in the practice-based portfolio increases in scope and complexity from year 1 to year 2 to year 3. Evidence presented includes written work, reflective accounts and critical incident analysis, as well as evidence of skills achievement for the designated skills for each module. Skills include clinical, transferable and cognitive elements. The portfolio is presented so that skills are integrated into theory, theory applied in practice and theory generated from practice experience.

The modified essay

An adaptation of the modified essay (Knox, 1980) is used in two of the modules in our BSc (Hons) in Nursing, one module in year 1 and one in year 2. From the learning outcomes for these two modules, a case scenario is selected that reflects a real practice situation likely to be encountered by students in clinical practice. The scenario is an evolving one that grows and develops. From the scenario, a series of questions are asked. These questions reflect the PBL process, for example: What do you know from this scenario? What additional information do you need? What hypotheses or suppositions can you make about the person in the scenario? What knowledge/information/understanding do you need to have to test these hypotheses? At different points in the questions, more information is injected into the scenario,

Table 8.1   Summary of assessments of a PBL programme

Year	Module	Module Title	Assessment	Weighting %
1	1	Beginning Life	**Theory–Practice Portfolio**	100
	2	Adolescence and Early Adult Life	**Theoretical:** Practice-based case study **Clinical:** Practice profile	75 25
	3	Adult Life	**Theoretical:** Modified essay **Clinical:** Practice profile	75 25
2	4	Later Life	**Theoretical:** Problem-based case study **Clinical:** Practice portfolio	75 25
	5	Health Breakdown and Interventions	**Theory–Practice Portfolio**	100
	6	Primary Healthcare Interventions	**Theoretical:** Modified essay **Clinical:** Practice portfolio	75 25
3	7	Secondary Healthcare Interventions	**Theoretical:** Problem-based case study **Clinical:** Practice portfolio	75 25
	8	Tertiary Healthcare Intervention	**Theory–Practice Portfolio**	100
	9	Towards Autonomous Practice	**Dissertation plus Practice Portfolio**	75 25

reflecting additional information received, test results made available, information from other healthcare professionals and so on. The students construct a problem-based answer to the scenario following the stages in the PBL tutorial process (Barrows, 1988). At the end, they come up with nursing actions that they would take for the person in the scenario with justification/evidence to support the suggested nursing actions.

In our BSc (Hons) programme, we give the scenario to the student group (learning set) prior to the actual writing of the essay. The group uses the problem-based tutorial process to work through the scenario, take responsibility for finding out information related to it and then share their information with each other. The writing up of the essay is, however, undertaken individually under normal examination conditions. In this way, the principle of learning in groups and sharing information, one of the key purposes of PBL, is maintained for part of the assessment process.

The problem-based case study

The case study is similar to any case study that a student may be required to submit during any nursing programme. However, for our programme, the instructions and parameters for completing the case study are written so that the student constructs the case study using a problem-based approach to a critical incident. The case study includes: presenting a critical incident scenario, identifying the issues related to the scenario, exploring the issues and presenting the student's evaluation of the situation, deductions and evidence-based decisions for nursing action. The case study also requires the student to reflect on the process and outcome.

These three approaches to assessment in the BSc (Hons) in Nursing are designed to assess a knowledge, skills and understanding of nursing, as well as to assess problem-solving, evidence-gathering, decision-making and reflection, all of which are key reasons for using a problem-based approach. Our ongoing evaluation of the programme includes evaluation of the assessment methods and their appropriateness.

Evaluation in PBL

At a recent multiprofessional conference, during a session on PBL, a medical registrar contributed to the ensuing discussion. He said that the evidence to date showed that there was little difference in the students at the end of a PBL programme, except that PBL graduates were possibly 'happier'. This comment was an illustration of how individual is the value each of us attaches to any outcome. It appeared that the value he placed on the outcome of happiness was insufficient to accept that PBL was a preferable means of learning to conventional, lecture-based ones. His evaluation of the situation was influenced by his own expectations and his personal priorities for education.

Evaluation, literally, means 'to take out the value' of something, and value can be considered to mean 'worth' or 'importance' (Quinn, 1988). It has become an essential part of any quality assurance mechanism, as the purpose of evaluation is to try to measure the success of the initiative. In education, this is to determine whether the activity being evaluated is significant to the students' learning. Was it *worth* the effort it took in terms of learning achieved? Was it *valued* by the students as an effective means to learning? Was it an *important* source of stimulus? Evaluation is inevitably subjective as value judgements are individual: what is important to one individual may not be to another. This makes not only the process of evaluation, but also action as a result of the evaluation a challenge. That famous saying, 'You can please some of the people all of the time and all of the people some of the time, but you cannot please all of the people all of the time' rings particularly true in this context. However, educationalists must try to make rational decisions on how to improve learning opportunities and how to please the majority; this necessitates a source of evidence on which to make these decisions. Programme evaluation by all major stakeholders is one source of evidence that can help in this process and that can help to make educational practice evidence based.

> Too often, educational innovations have been adopted without proper assessment of their merits. Innovations that are effective on a small scale with dedicated teachers have been found to fail when implemented on a large scale with teachers who are less enthusiastic. (Albanese and Mitchell, 1993, p. 53)

Evaluation is an important element of curriculum design in any type of educational programme. Margetson (1995) suggests that this is especially true in PBL, in which evaluation should be integrated into the programme structure to be consistent with the very nature of PBL. This section will review some of the published evidence in relation to PBL in order to consider types of evaluation that can be used. It will also provide a case study of evaluation methods currently being implemented in a preregistration midwifery PBL programme.

Literature review on evaluation methods being used in PBL

The literature available that evaluates PBL comes primarily from medical education programmes as this is where PBL has its longest history, having been initiated at McMaster University in the late 1960s (Berkson, 1993). In three sources in particular, results from a large number of programmes are examined in meta-analysis-type reviews, providing considerable data upon which to reflect and try to determine the value of PBL. The emphasis in this type of review is on quantity in that there is an attempt to measure, quantify and generalise from the findings of a variety of evaluative studies. The data collected are both 'hard' (for example, the results of assessments, the ability to undertake effective clinical examination, the recall of facts, and costs) and 'soft' (for example, student and staff satisfaction); some (for example, trying to determine the critical abilities of two groups of students) cross the two paradigms. The methodology of systematic review is, however, profoundly based in the scientific paradigm, in which quantity is considered to be the most convincing parameter.

Albanese and Mitchell (1993) examined the English language international literature from 1972 to 1992 in an attempt critically to examine the effectiveness of PBL. They reported on 17 studies of medical PBL programmes from nine different universities in the USA, Canada, Australia and The Netherlands. Their conclusions are that PBL is more nurturing and enjoyable than traditional lecture-based programmes, and that PBL graduates perform as well, and sometimes better, on both clinical examinations and faculty evaluations. Also, lecturers generally enjoy teaching using PBL. However, PBL students did, in a few instances, score lower on basic science examinations, and they perceived themselves to be less well prepared in basic sciences than their counterparts on conventional programmes. They were also found to engage in backward reasoning rather than the forward reasoning that experts engage in, and there were gaps in their cognitive knowledge base.

Costs were also felt to be worthy of consideration as the small-group techniques used in PBL can have resource implications. This review integrates a number of different sources of evaluation exploring student and staff opinion, assessment results, performance in practice, style of reasoning and costs. The authors concluded at the end of the review that, despite many positive results from PBL programmes, these should not be implemented on a wide scale basis without further research. Their main concern appeared to relate to the poorer results from PBL programmes, leading to the conclusion that these should not be implemented on a wide scale basis without further research.

Berkson (1993) also reviewed medical education PBL programmes, 11 in total. Using the results on assessment as the measure, the academic achievements of the students, on these 11 programmes, showed that in 5 cases the results were equivalent on PBL and traditional curricula, in 3 cases the results were slightly better with PBL and in 3 cases the results were slightly/marginally worse with PBL. On this basis, the author concludes that the PBL graduate is difficult to distinguish from a traditionally educated counterpart. She also suggests that PBL can be stressful to both faculty and students (this conclusion being arrived at as the result of one study that the author acknowledges to be flawed by the poor response rate of traditional students) and that it may be unreasonably costly (this being, once again, based on a single study). Most of the evaluation methods used in this review related to quantitative data, and the conclusion reached was swayed by priority being given to 'hard' outcomes.

Vernon and Blake (1993) conducted 5 separate meta-analyses on 35 studies representing 19 institutions. Their conclusions indicate that students evaluate PBL programmes more highly, the faculty's attitudes towards PBL are most positive, and students' mood, class attendance and academic progress are all improved with PBL. There is an integration of qualitative and quantitative elements in this review, but the main emphasis relates to the positive experiences of participants.

Apart from these meta-analyses, a number of individual reports provide additional evaluative data regarding PBL, some of which also relate primarily to the satisfaction and experience of participants. Kaufman and Mann (1996) compared the perceptions of two cohorts of students at the end of their second year in medical school; one group had followed a traditional, lecture-based curriculum and the other a PBL one. The students in the PBL curriculum rated their course significantly higher than did students on the conventional course on 11 out of 12 items, which included higher-level thinking, managing information, stimulating self-directed learning and overall satisfaction. The one item that they rated lower was the learning of details. This lower learning of details was also found to be the case by Martensen *et al.* (1992); however, the PBL students rated all of the other dimensions evaluated more positively than did those students undertaking a similar 9-week course on the musculoskeletal system with a conventional format. Pinto Pereira *et al.* (1993) reported that PBL students find the approach stimulating as well as demanding. Moore *et al.* (1994) reported that students at Harvard Medical School found their preclinical medical education using PBL to be more challenging and satisfying than their counterparts in the traditional curriculum.

All of these studies have evaluated the students' perceptions of PBL. An example of one study focusing more on measurable outcomes is reported by Lewis and Buckley (1992), who found no difference in the assessment outcomes for students on PBL programmes, but did find that they were better prepared to learn 'deeply'.

It would seem that this review of some of the evaluative literature leads us to the same conclusion held by the medical registrar at the PBL presentation mentioned at the beginning of this section of the chapter. The 'hard' outcomes (for example, student assessment results) show that there is little difference between the PBL graduate and one from a conventional educational programme in medicine. However, the 'soft' outcomes relating to satisfaction and 'happiness' seem to indicate that students prefer this method of learning. There are some points, however, that possibly require further evaluation, for example the learning of detail and the cost of implementing PBL.

The point of examining the findings in these reports in the context of this chapter is to consider the types of evaluation used. Evaluation methods will be determined by those evaluating; the questions they ask will be decided by their own priorities. There are a variety of methods of evaluation available, none being right or wrong, but different methods will provide different information, which can be used by curriculum-planners to improve the learning experience of students.

Types of evaluation: a case study

The two paradigms in research/evaluation – quantitative and qualitative – can be related to two approaches to curriculum: product and process (Kelly, 1989). The emphasis on hard outcomes means that the focus is mainly on the final outcome of the educational programme, less interest being devoted to how the students get there. In contrast, the quality of the process of learning can be considered to be of more importance, taking into account outcomes that may not be measurable through assessment and pass/fail rates. Both the process and the product have significant roles to play in effective education, and both can feature in programme evaluation. Fisher (1991) claims that there is a third dimension to evaluation, that of input, in which the plans and objectives of the programme are examined. If we accept that all three of these are important elements, a flow diagram of the evaluation of any programme, including a PBL one, can be created. This model needs to be set in the overall context of the programme delivery, which will include both professional and university/institutional requirements for level, standards and competence.

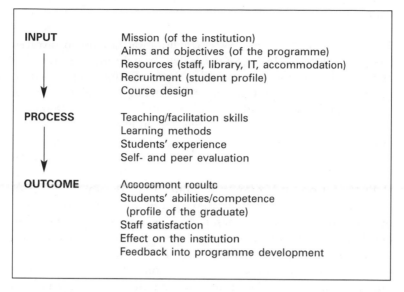

INPUT	Mission (of the institution)
	Aims and objectives (of the programme)
	Resources (staff, library, IT, accommodation)
	Recruitment (student profile)
	Course design
PROCESS	Teaching/facilitation skills
	Learning methods
	Students' experience
	Self- and peer evaluation
OUTCOME	Assessment results
	Students' abilities/competence
	(profile of the graduate)
	Staff satisfaction
	Effect on the institution
	Feedback into programme development

Figure 8.1   A flow diagram of the evaluation of a programme

At Thames Valley University in 1997, the preregistration midwifery curriculum was revalidated using a PBL approach. The curriculum development team reviewed the evidence in relation to the effectiveness of the method in general and were convinced that it could make a valid contribution to midwifery education, although there was virtually nothing in the literature about its use in midwifery. As it appeared that this would be the first PBL midwifery programme in England, the team felt that it was vital for the programme to be rigorously evaluated to provide evidence for other curriculum-planners in midwifery. With that aim in mind, evaluation using the above model began with the first intake in September 1997. It was felt that a combination of both qualitative and quantitative data would help to present a complete picture, so the evaluation methods being used are diverse.

Context

The context in which the new curriculum was developed involved a large Institute of Health Sciences that brought together two pre-existing midwifery schools. Both had been offering preregistration midwifery; one school offered an 18-month degree-level programme for qualified nurses, and the other both 3-year and 18-month diploma programmes. The curriculum planning team analysed the evaluations of the three different programmes as a starting point for deciding what was already working well. A literature search was conducted to bring together issues of professional legislation (UKCC, European Community and ENB recommendations), research on effective midwifery education and topical issues from practice such as evidence-based approaches to care. The team decided that PBL would integrate these pertinent concepts into an appropriate learning method for prospective midwives.

Prior to the first intake of students on the PBL programme, questionnaires were distributed to the midwife assessors who support students during their practice experience. The questions related to the expected outcomes of a PBL programme; we wanted to know how well the midwives thought the existing students were doing in relation to lifelong learning skills, using research in practice, self-directed study and communication skills. The background information helped to complete the context in which the new programme would sit. The truth was that the majority of respondents felt that the existing students were already doing quite well.

Input

The university's mission is a powerful one that incorporates the wish to open access to higher education with a student-centred approach to learning. This appears to be in keeping with the PBL philosophy and is therefore an appropriate initial input into the curriculum. The aims and objectives of the programme are, obviously, driven by professional legislation and guidance, but the curriculum planning team wanted this programme to prepare midwives not only to be able to fulfil statutory responsibilities, but also to be motivated and skilled to drive the profession forward in post-*Changing Childbirth* (DoH, 1993) days. It seemed reasonable that an active, student-centred method of learning would help to develop midwives supportive of woman-centred practice. Both the mission and aims/objectives are reasonably immovable, but the wider expectations require observation of the students, once qualified, to determine whether they have developed the anticipated philosophy for practice.

The resources available for students on the programme are far ranging. The most important are probably the women and babies, as well as the midwives with whom they practise under supervision. Fifty per cent of the programme is delivered in practice; students are directed to use these resources to help them to learn from the experiences of both professionals and women having babies. Additional resources include the learning resource centres with books, journals, databases and videos, the praxis laboratories with models and interactive learning packages (a developing source), and tutorial staff who are available through the link teacher network and in 'fixed resource sessions'. These sessions are currently being evaluated by students using questionnaires, the other resources being evaluated through end of semester programme evaluations conducted in the learning sets (8–10 students).

Students are recruited to the programme via first an application and then an interview. During the interviews, there are group discussions in which students are shown two photographs that will 'trigger' thinking. The photographs are of a tiered lecture theatre full of students and a small tutorial group, students being asked to discuss the two approaches to learning. Once the discussion is complete, providing an ideal opportunity for the observing tutorial staff to determine the communication skills of applicants, the students are told about the PBL approach to learning in the programme. The interview is perceived as much as an opportunity for them to decide whether our approach suits them as it is for us to decide their suitability. This approach to recruitment is being evaluated in order to determine whether we are preparing students effectively for the approach to learning.

The overall course design is based on the Maastricht approach to PBL (Schmidt, 1983), in which 'triggers' are used to 'activate learning'. As midwifery is an occupation in which women are supported through a normal physiological process, the lecturing team found it difficult to accept the concept of basing learning on problems. For the vast majority of women, having a baby is not a problem; to create midwives who believed that their role was to solve problems for women was contrary to the underlying philosophy. It was therefore agreed that stimuli would be provided to students that helped them to focus their learning in relevant areas rather than constructing problems for which there was a 'right' answer. The triggers are currently being evaluated through nominal group technique at the end of each tutorial cycle to determine their effectiveness in stimulating learning.

Process

The preparation of tutorial staff is felt to be a crucial component of the success of a PBL programme (Mitchell, 1988; Murrell, 1996). The team of midwifery lecturers at Thames Valley University were already skilled at interactive learning, commonly using group-work, seminars, role-play, debates and so on. However, PBL moves beyond these activities in that the teacher is no longer in the position of control over student learning in the same way as on conventional programmes. In order to prepare staff for the change to PBL, initial staff development opportunities were provided (as weekly sessions over a 6-month period) to the lecturers who were facilitating the learning sets; this process is carrying on as new issues arise from their actually participating in PBL. The lecturers have been interviewed by the evaluation team in order to determine their perspectives on the effectiveness of PBL. They are also completing reflective diaries that will provide more insight into their experiences in this different approach to teaching (cf. Chapter 3).

The students' perceptions of the programme may be the single most important element to evaluate. The students on this programme had no experience of PBL prior to the course commencing, and there has been a mixed response to date. Data are being collected from end of semester evaluations using a standard University evaluation form and interviews with students, and via the trigger evaluations (students often raising issues to do with the method along with those to do with the actual triggers). These sources can be triangulated to give a well-rounded picture of student impression.

Students are encouraged to evaluate their own effectiveness in relation to three elements at the end of each tutorial cycle, as suggested by Barrows (1988). These three issues are: the ability to problem-solve, self-directed learning skill and contribution to the working of the group. This informal evaluation helps the students to develop their skills of self-assessment and prepares them for a summative assessment in the final semester, that of a peer review. The students' results on the peer review may be a particularly helpful aspect of the programme evaluation as success may indicate that PBL has had a positive impact on the ability to share learning in a supportive and critical manner.

Outcome

The results of assessments, both in theory and in practice, provide another measure of success, including a comparison of passes, referrals and failures with students on previous programmes, as well as classification of degrees. Students will be interviewed on completion of the programme. It will be interesting to see whether there is any difference in the number who actually go into and stay in midwifery practice, as the learning throughout the programme is contextual to the profession rather than divided into subject specialist areas as was the case in the past.

Staff satisfaction will be evaluated in the interviews with staff, but also can be seen on a day-to-day basis in the discussions happening over lunch and at team meetings. The researcher leading the evaluation has been attending the staff development sessions to keep records of the concerns expressed and achievements shared. It is fair to say that the change to PBL has been a challenge for staff, but the enthusiasm displayed in terms of wanting to 'get it right' has been very reassuring.

The effects on the institution will be evaluated by determining how widespread PBL becomes as a result of the evaluation of the midwifery programme. Programmes in other areas will be able to learn from the evaluation and feed this knowledge into future curriculum development. Recruitment to the PBL programme will be another measure of success; as the method becomes more understood and the approach disseminated in the midwifery community, there may be an impact on numbers applying for the course.

Conclusion

PBL presents unique challenges with regard to the assessment of student achievement and the evaluation of the programme. There is an imperative within PBL to obtain evaluative data in order to make evidence-based decisions about programme development. The literature offers a wide range of assessment and evaluation methods that are compatible and congruent with PBL. The primary principle remains, however, that when PBL is introduced, the assessment techniques and evaluation methods must reflect the underlying principles and intentions of PBL. At Thames Valley University, we are using a variety of these techniques and methods to assess student achievement and evaluate our programmes. This will provide us with useful evidence for other institutions that may be considering PBL in the future.

References

Albanese, M A and Mitchell, S (1993) Problem-based Learning: A Review of the Literature on its Outcomes and Implementation Issues, *Academica Medica*, **68**(1): 52–81.

Barrows, H S (1988) *The Tutorial Process*, Springfield, IL: Southern Illinois University School of Medicine.

Berkson, L (1993) Problem-based Learning: Have Expectations Been Met?, *Academic Medicine*, **68**(10): S79–S87.

Boud, D J (1988) Assessment in Problem-based Learning, *Assessment and Evaluation in Higher Education*, **13**: 87–91.

Department of Health (1993) *Changing Childbirth: Report of the Expert Maternity Group*, London: HMSO.

Engel, C (1991) Not Just a Method but a Way of Learning. In Boud, D and Feletti, G (eds), *The Challenge of Problem-based Learning*, London: Kogan Page.

Feletti, G (1980) Reliability and Validity Studies on Modified Essay Questions, *Journal of Medical Education*, **55**(11): 931–4.

Feletti, G, Saunders, N and Smith, A (1983) Comprehensive Assessment of Final Year Medical Student Performance Based on Undergraduate Programme Objectives, *Lancet*, **2**: 34–7.

Fisher, L A (1991) Evaluating the Impact of Problem-based Learning on the Institution and on the Faculty. In Boud, D and Feletti, G (eds), *The Challenge of Problem-based Learning*, London: Kogan Page.

Hodgkin, K and Knox, J D E (1975) *Problem Centred Learning*, Edinburgh: Churchill Livingstone.

Kaufman, D M and Mann, K V (1996) Evaluating Problem-based Learning: Students' Perceptions about their Courses in Problem-based Learning and Conventional Curricula, *Academic Medicine*, **71**(1): 552–4.

Kelly, A V (1989) *The Curriculum: Theory And Practice*, London: Paul Chapman.

Knox, J D E (1980) How To Use Modified Essay Questions, *Medical Teacher*, **2**(1): 20–4.

Lewis, M E and Buckley A, (1992) The Role of Evaluation. In Kong, M and Mellsop, G W (eds), Development of a Problem-based Learning Programme within a Traditional School of Medicine, *Annals of Community-oriented Education*, **5**: 223–34.

Margetson, D (1991) Why is Problem-based Learning a Challenge? In Boud, D and Feletti, G (eds) *The Challenge of Problem-based Learning*, London: Kogan Page, pp. 42–50.

Margetson, D (1995) The Role of Evaluation. In Alavi, C (ed.) *Problem-based Learning in a Health Sciences Curriculum*, London: Routledge.

Martensen, D, Eriksson, H and Ingelman-Sundberg, M (1985) Medical Chemistry: Evaluation of Active and Problem-oriented Teaching Methods, *Medical Education*, **19**: 34–42.

Martensen, D, Myklebust, R and Stalsberg H (1992) Implementing Problem-based Learning within a Lecture-dominated Curriculum: Results and Processes, *Teaching and Learning in Medicine*, **4**: 233–7.

Mitchell, G (1988) Problem-based Learning in Medical Schools: A New Approach, *Medical Teacher*, **10**(1): 57–67.

Moore, G T, Block, S D, Briggs Style, C and Mitchell, R (1994) The Influence of the New Pathway Curriculum on Harvard Medical Students, *Academic Medicine* **69**: 983–9.

Murrell, J P (1996) Incorporating Problem-based Learning: Striving Towards Woman-centred Care, *British Journal of Midwifery*, **4**(9): 479.

Norman, G (1989) Reliability and Validity of Some Cognitive Measures of Clinical Reasoning, *Teaching and Learning in Medicine*, **1**(4): 194–9.

Norman, G (1991) What Should Be Assessed? In Boud, D and Feletti, G (eds), *The Challenge of Problem-based Learning*, London: Kogan Page.

Norman, G R and Schmidt, H G (1992) The Psychological Basis of Problem-based Learning: A Review of the Evidence, *Academic Medicine*, **67**: 557–65.

Painvin, C, Neufeld, V R and Norman, G R (1979) The Triple Jump Exercise – a Structured Measure of Problem-solving and Self-directed Learning, *Proceedings of the 18th Conference of Research in Medical Education*, November, Washington DC.

Pallie, W and Carr, D H (1987) The McMaster Medical Education Philosophy in Theory, Practice and Historical Perspective, *Medical Teacher*, **9**(1): 59–71.

Pinto Pereira, L, Telang, B, Butler, K and Joseph, S (1993) Preliminary Evaluation of a New Curriculum – Incorporation of Problem Based Learning (PBL) into the Traditional Format, *Medical Teacher*, **15**(4): 351–64.

Powles, A, Wintrip, N, Neufeld, V, Wakefield, J, Coates, G and Burrows J (1981) The 'Triple Jump' Exercise: Further Studies of an Evaluative Technique, Proceedings of the 20th annual Conference of Research in Medical Education, Washington, DC, November.

Quinn, F (1988) *Principles and Practices of Nurse Education*, London: Chapman & Hall.

Rezler, A G (1989) Self-assessment in Problem-based Learning, *Medical Teacher*, **11**(2): 151–6.

Schmidt, H G (1983) Problem Based Learning: Rationale and Description, *Medical Education*, **17**: 11–16.

Silén, C (1998) Understanding and Qualitative Assessment, Paper presented at the 6th annual Improving Student Learning Symposium, University of Brighton, 7–9 September.

Swanson, D (1987) A Measurement Framework for Performance-based Tests. In Hart, I and Harden, R (eds) *Further Developments in Assessing Clinical Competence*, Montreal: Heal Publications.

Swanson, D, Norcini, J and Grosso, L (1987) Assessment of Clinical Competence: Written and Computer-based Simulations, *Assessment and Evaluation in Higher Education*, **12**: 220–46.

Swanson, D, Case S and Van der Vleuten, C P M (1991) Strategies for Student Assessment. In Boud, D and Feletti, G (eds), *The Challenge of Problem-based Learning*, London: Kogan Page.

Vernon D T A and Blake R L (1993) The Psychological Basis of Problem-based Learning: A Review of the Evidence, *Academic Medicine*, **67**: 557–65.

9

An Educational Model for Preparation for Practice?

Iain Burns and Sally Glen

Healthcare organisations are now seeking a multiskilled, responsive, adaptable workforce who are prepared to be lifelong learners, adapting and changing as required by the organisation. The scope of modern nursing is still evolving. Just as nursing practice adapts to changes in healthcare provision, so too must nurse education if it is to remain 'current' (Boettcher, 1994). If nurses are to be prepared for a pivotal role in the care of people in the twenty-first century, nurse education has to develop innovative and creative initiatives to meet the needs of the citizens of the region served (Berkley, 1992). Nurse educationalists thus have a responsibility to encourage and develop nurses who can respond proactively to the rapidly changing healthcare environment and the requirements of demanding healthcare consumers (a key theme of this book).

To meet this challenge, nurse educators must pass two basic tests. The first is how well they equip nurses to apply their knowledge in contexts beyond the bounds of their formal educational experience, and the second, how well they motivate and equip nurses and midwives to continue learning throughout their professional lives. The passing of these two basic tests may require a new model of nurse education to mitigate 'academic drift', which is often regarded as a distinctive and persistent feature of higher education (Glen, 1995). Nurse educationalists will be required to show that their programmes of education avoid this trap. These programmes must not only be cost-effective, innovative and up to date, but also produce the desired outcome in terms of a nurse who is ready to meet the challenges of an ever-changing health service. It has been recognised that, in many cases, educationalists in all fields have been, in the words of Margetson (1994, p. 5), 'hanging on to curricula which have lost their point'. Similarly, the WHO also recognises that the education of health professionals does not always meet societal needs (WHO, 1993). The WHO (1993) advocates the widespread introduction of PBL into health professional education. This is in part due to the fact that PBL is offered by many educationalists as a solution to some of the current problems within professional education, and to the growing body of research and literature that is providing evidence of the value of (PBL) curricula in the education of healthcare professionals (cf. Chapter 2). One of the problems is, of course, 'academic drift'.

'Academic drift'

Nursing education is now clearly part of the higher education sector. The effects of the all-pervasive ethos of the university might be far reaching in nursing education, and not necessarily beneficial in all instances. Squires (1990, p. 18) argues that the academic theoretical orientation can yield benefits in terms of knowledge and academic status, but:

> It can also produce a reaction which attacks the increasing irrelevance or distortion of such studies. Practitioners, it is claimed, have their heads filled with jargon and are no longer adequately prepared for the 'real world'.

Similarly, Cohen (1985, p. 7) argues:

> The demand for academic respectability changes the context and the method. The object of the training, the production of skilled effective professional workers recedes, and the training of critical knowledgeable scholars take precedence.

Helping students to acquire a sound theoretical knowledge of nursing work and its value is clearly an important aim for preregistration programmes. However, of equal importance are opportunities to practise skills in order to develop 'know-how', that is, the knowledge of how to *do* the work of nursing (cf. Chapter 8). May *et al.* (1997), for example, refer to one student's awareness of an element of the theory–practice dilemma: 'I know what I should do, I just don't know how to do it.' This would be supported by Schön (1983, p. 16) who argued that although professionals are recognised in society for their professional knowledge, the knowledge gained by professionals does not, however, always enable them to cope with the 'complexity, uncertainty, instability, uniqueness and value conflicts perceived as central to the world of professional practice' (a key theme of this book).

An additional difficulty is that there is no one agreed template of performance or skills that might be used as a 'measure' of baseline competence. This situation contributes to problems of validity and reliability in assessment, as well as to the design of studies that seek to examine performance following registration. Not only is the scope of competence unclear, but it also shifts, a feature evident in nursing at the beginning of the millennium and one that can cause difficulties for employers and educators. Eraut raises important questions about the extent to which preregistration common foundation and branch programmes of nurse education are responsive to change within roles and able to prepare nurses for the range of competences, both general and specific, that employers need:

> In professions (or specialism within professions) where work is relatively homogenous, there will be little confusion between statements of general and specific competence because the one can be inferred from the other. But in professions or specialisms where the work is relatively heterogeneous and one professional may handle a completely different set of situations from that of another, general statements become rather dangerous. The client or prospective employer will need a profile of specific competencies which clearly demonstrates those aspects of the job in which each professional is competent. However, this nice tidy picture ignores the fact that in many occupations the nature of the work is changing quite rapidly, not only as a result of technical change but also as a result of social change and institutional change. (Eraut, 1994, p. 165)

The questions that educationalists and nurses must ask themselves are: 'What knowledge and skills do nurses need to practise?', 'How do we help students gain the appropriate knowledge and skills for effective practice?', and 'How do we facilitate the development of lifelong learning skills in our students?' It is essential, in considering the answer to these issues, that nursing education takes cognisance of 'the messy, real world of nursing practice' (Miller, 1985 p. 420). Decision-making in clinical nursing practice is, in reality, more often composed of contextually defined value judgements. Greenwood (1993), for example, distinguishes between the practice of nursing and the applicability of the scientific paradigm to such practice. This view reflects an Aristotelian practical view of the theory–practice relationship in which practice is seen as a moral activity requiring judgement, wisdom and prudence in complex changing situations. The task of theory is to make morally defensible decisions and choices by developing the art of practical deliberations among practitioners to facilitate the improvement of practice.

In the UK, nursing work-based learning has long been valued and considered to be of equal importance to university-based learning. The value of a long history of experience in this area should not be underestimated. Nurse educators could learn much from the 'academic drift' of professions such as teaching, the law, social work and architecture. There is a feeling in teaching, for example, that the education of teachers was hijacked by academics in the 1970s and early 80s, with adverse results for practice. In the 1990s, we witnessed a substantial shift away from university-based professional preparation to school-based preparation. Theoretical ideas cannot usually be applied 'off the shelf': their implications have to be worked out and thought through (Eraut, 1994). Criticisms such as these have led to a reconceptualisation of the theory–practice dichotomy, and of partnership in training and education between the 'trainers' and practising professionals. There is a need to achieve academic and clinical credibility. Alternative models of professional education from other professions and other countries provide some ideas.

The integration of theory and practice

As higher education has been used more and more as an entry route by professions seeking higher status, much has been heard about the relationship between theory and practice. Like theory, 'practice' cannot be considered to be one single entity. It may involve a client, or other professionals, or it may not involve another person as such. An example of the latter might be the assimilation of the contents of a client file and adding to it in ways useful to other readers. Being critical about professional practice therefore needs to be unpacked, analysed and properly developed in the different fields of professional practice. Similarly, some nurses use the term 'theory' variously and uncritically, sometimes to denote teaching carried out in the classroom, sometimes to differentiate knowledge learned in the classroom from knowledge learned in practice (Mackenzie, 1994), at other times to refer to any knowledge useful in understanding or providing care, or to published research, product evaluation or literature reviews (Cody, 1994). Some nurses do seem to have a clear understanding and assert that their practice is research based, yet they nevertheless behave differently when working with patients, suggesting a distinction between 'espoused theory' and 'theory in practice' (NHS Executive, 1998) (cf. Chapter 6).

Not surprisingly, there is a wealth of nursing literature that has attempted to reconcile the apparent divergence between theory and practice. The hoped-for resolution of this apparent dilemma has been seen to lie along a spectrum between bringing theory to practice – the lecturer/practitioner role (Champion, 1992; Lathlean, 1992; Glen and Clark, 1999) – and bringing practice to theory: the critical incident (Smith and Russell, 1991). Eraut (1985, 1994) advocates a close partnership between the decontextualised knowledge taught by university staff and knowledge in context. Students' and practitioners' contextual knowledge is advanced by collaborative research between educationalists and practitioners. In other words, the theory–practice relationship should be conceptualised as a sociological rather than an epistemological issue.

We have entered an era in which, in all professional fields, importance is attached to the idea of partnership in training and education between the 'trainers' and practising professionals. The moving of nursing education into the university setting may have resulted in its distancing from the clinical setting (Varcoe and Cresswell, 1993). The different values and perspectives of education and service may result in competing educational objectives and service requirements (Elkan and Robinson, 1993; Walsh, 1997). A reconciliation of competing imperatives may be a necessary condition for the greater integration of the theory and practice. Furthermore, if clinical staff are constrained in providing the right kind of experience and support for students, it has been argued that alternatives must be sought (Prowse, 1996). Schools and departments of nursing and midwifery should thus support the development of clinically focused programmes and modules in partnership with service colleagues.

Successful educational and practising professionals' partnerships go some way to addressing the integration of theory and practice (Cornes, 1998). Such partnerships would provide, for example, greater opportunities for nurse lecturers to utilise clinical areas in order to upgrade their knowledge and to familiarise themselves with new technology and trends in client/patient care. In addition, nurse lecturers can, through easier access to the clinical areas, have greater opportunities to maintain and develop their own clinical skills. Alternatively, the partnership can offer clinical practitioners easier access to the lecturers, who are more conversant with research findings that might have relevance to nursing practice in order to enhance the quality of client/patient care. In reality, clinical practitioners find it extremely difficult, if not impossible, to remain professionally up to date in all areas of nursing, particularly specialist ones (Fay, 1986).

Eraut (1985) seeks to find a role for higher education other than the transmission of generalisable knowledge to professional communities. More recently, Eraut (1994) has suggested that higher education should extend its role from that of creator and transmitter of knowledge to individuals and professional communities. This would involve recognising that much knowledge creation takes place outside the higher education system, but is nevertheless limited by the absence of appropriate support structures and the prevailing action orientation of practical contexts. Hence, Eraut suggests that higher education institutions and professional communities should establish closer relations and assume joint responsibility for knowledge creation, development and dissemination. Some joint ventures might be:

- Collaborative research projects into the acquisition and development of important areas of professional knowledge and know-how.
- Problem-oriented seminars for groups of researchers and mid-career professionals, including, when relevant, members of other professions.
- The joint ownership, development and implementation of post-registration modules and programmes.

The improvement in both pre- and postregistration nurse education is likely to be dependent on a broader view of what constitutes professional knowledge and know-how, more information about how nurses develop such knowledge and a deeper consideration of how nurses learn. In the university, knowledge is enshrined and encoded in predesigned curricula and organisational structures; in the world outside in clinical practice, knowledge is everywhere, waiting for practitioners to create their own value from it. If the integration of theory and practice is important, a reallocation of resources is required to shift the focus of investment away from the classroom to the clinical/practice component of education programmes.

A relationship between theory and practice may be impossible (cf. Chapters 1 and 6). However, in May *et al.*'s (1997) study, students were found to 'back off' from exploring gaps between theory and practice for fear of being seen as critical. Practice development can benefit from the understanding that practice may lag behind theory, but that theory itself may not reflect current practice. A newly qualified nurse who had such an understanding would need freedom to continue to question, albeit in a supportive environment that encouraged discussion. May *et al.* (1997) go so far as to suggest that the Project 2000 programmes contain the potential solution to the problem of the theory–practice gap through providing opportunities for and developing skills in reflective discussion. Students should be offered the notions of grounded theory, practical principles and craft knowledge, which are directly derived from, and readily applicable to, practice (Eraut, 1995). Within nurse education, the message has been very similar (Cornes, 1998). For example, the UKCC document 'A Statement of Strategic Intent' (UKCC, 1994) emphasised the essential need for collaboration at every level in the provision of both pre- and postregistration nurse education. The document agreed that such partnership would place the students at the centre of the learning experience within a framework that is practice led, research based and employment focused. This theme was re-emphasised in Fitness for Practice (UKCC, 1999) and Making a Difference (DoH, 1999).

Towards a new model of nursing education

The process of becoming a nurse involves learning to handle cases quickly and efficiently, and this may be accomplished by reducing the range of possible ways of thinking about them to manageable proportions. This leads to an intuitive reliance on certain communal practitioners' concepts (Buchmann, 1980), while apparently more valid theoretical ideas get consigned to 'storage' and never get retrieved. The functional relevance of a piece of theoretical knowledge depends less on its presumed validity than on the ability and willingness of nurses to use it. This is mainly determined by individual nurses and their practice context, but it is also affected by the way in which the knowledge is introduced and linked to their professional concerns.

This way of conceiving of nursing practice has profound implications for nursing education. It implies that a curriculum that first offers students theoretical components, and then expects them to put the theory 'into practice' in the practical situation, is misconceived. Campbell and Jackson (1992) point out the limitations of the scientific model of nursing as a basis of learner instruction and state that new curricula must deal with the practical, immediate issues of nursing as a *lived* experience. The disciplines are used, as Chandler (1991) suggests, not for 'application' to practice but to question the legitimacy and effectiveness of nursing work and behaviour. Some nurse educators, however, continue to subscribe to a highly theoretical approach to developing diploma and degree curricula. Professional knowledge is seen to consist of a theoretical understanding of ideas drawn from disciplines such as physiology, psychology, philosophy and sociology, plus 'knowing how' to apply them in particular practical situations. Practitioners thus acquire theoretical knowledge from the disciplines, often taught in separation from each other, and are then expected to apply it in practice. Such an approach can lead to a fragmented rather than a holistic approach to care, or to a view that the knowledge is not perceived as relevant to practice (Acton *et al.*, 1992; Charlesworth *et al.*, 1992). Traditional lecturer-based courses have therefore been criticised for an overreliance on subjects against the development of enquiry skills, a failure to deal with the issues faced by students in professional practice and a poor development of team-working (Boud and Feletti, 1991).

If the objective of nursing education is the development of a critically thinking reflective nurse, the nursing community must review its present teaching strategies, outcomes and existing educational philosophy in terms of teacher–student relationships, valued forms of knowing and learning, and society's expectations of the registered nurse. What is needed is a new model of nursing education. There is a need to build on the strengths of both traditions. The best must be retained while continuing to strive for improvement and innovation. The concern about the shift in emphasis towards the academic base of nursing at the expense of the practical base has been noted in Chapter 1. Yet the two are not incompatible, and it has been suggested that the best of the apprenticeship model can be adopted and built upon (Morse, 1996).

Nursing education should be seen to be, in effect, an analysis of both the liberal and vocational educational traditions. From the liberal tradition comes the notion of commitment to an extensive knowledge base (with the implication of an aspiration to its concomitant status associations); from the vocational tradition comes a commitment to mastering technical skills, community service and earning a living from the practice of the occupation. It is not a reliable aim to produce a technician or a professional. Nursing is grounded in practice, and with this in mind, educational principles and procedures should foster critical thinking and problem-solving. The implementation of such a model would demand that the curriculum be organised around PBL. PBL offers particular attraction as a context for multiprofessional education as it promotes co-operation as opposed to competition between participants (Brandon and Majundar, 1997).

In adopting a PBL model for curriculum design, the students are presented with a 'problem situation'. The emphasis is on encouraging the students to use their existing knowledge, a deficiency of traditional passive teaching methods (Amos and White,

1998), and explore 'what needs to be known to address and improve a particular situation' (Boud and Feletti, 1997, p. 16) (cf. Chapters 2 and 7).

Nursing is a practice-based profession, so the knowledge gained must help nurses to engage in and develop their practice. Nurse education must, as Townsend (1990, p. 61) suggests, be based on a curriculum that is 'grounded in and derived from that practice'. PBL is advocated as a model of adult education that allows this to happen. It is a method that enables students to explore what Boud and Feletti (1997) term 'real-life' situations, with the emphasis on problem-solving and team-work. Students are therefore able to develop educational and practical skills that enable them to cope with an ever-changing world in which lifelong learning is essential.

PBL is seen as a way to ensure that deeper learning, which is relevant to practice, actually happens (cf. Chapter 8). Doring *et al.* (1995) see PBL as a way of ensuring that students become fully involved in the learning process, while Townsend (1990), among others, points out that the problem situations or triggers utilised within the PBL component of the curriculum are drawn from practice, and the solutions or knowledge required to deal with the issues must therefore be directly related to the practice situation. This also ensures that PBL offers a more 'integrated approach to learning' and that the learning that takes place 'will enable the student to approach care delivery in a holistic manner' (Williams, 1998 p. 15). This premise is also supported by Bawden (1997). In discussing PBL within a curriculum for professional agriculturists, Bawden noted that there is in a traditional curriculum a 'fragmentation of effort' that works against the development of skills needed for today's professional practice. PBL, on the other hand, ensures that students 'learn how to improve situations across an enormous range of complexity through their involvement in real world projects' (Bawden, 1997, p. 331).

Conclusion

The perceived inadequacies of both university-based courses and traditional work-based courses have necessitated the adoption, implementation and growing acceptance of new and alternative practices such as PBL. PBL facilitates the development of links between theory and clinical practice in a meaningful way, and could provide the framework for the revolution in nursing education to occur as a result of its integration into higher education. In essence, it provides a new model of nursing education.

References

Acton, L, Gough, P, McCormack, B (1992) The Clinical Nurse Tutor Debate, *Nursing Times*, **88**(32): 38–40.

Amos, E and White, M J (1998) Teaching Tools: Problem-based Learning, *Nurse Educator*, **23**(2): 11–14.

Bawden, R (1997) Towards a Praxis of Situation Improving. In Boud, D and Feletti, G (eds), *The Challenge of Problem-based Learning* (2nd edn), London: Kogan Page.

Berkley, T W (1992) Perform and Re-structuring in Nurse Education: A Necessity for Nursing Future in Florida, *The Florida Nurse*, (March).

Boettcher, J H (1996) Nurse Practice Centres in Academia: An Emerging Subsystem, *Journal of Nurse Education*, **35**(2): 63–8.

Boud, D and Feletti, G (1991) *The Challenge of Problem-based Learning*, London: Kogan Page.

Boud, D and Feletti, G (1997) *The Challenge of Problem-based Learning* (2nd edn), London: Kogan Page.

Brandon, J E and Majundar, B (1997) An Introduction and Evaluation of Problem-based Learning in Health Profession's Education, *Family Community Health*, **20**(1): 1–15.

Buchmann, A (1980) *Practitioners' Concepts: An Inquiry into the Wisdom of Practice*, Occasional Paper No. 29, Michigan: Michigan State University, Institute for Research and Training.

Campbell, M L and Jackson, N S (1992) Learning to Nurse: Plans, Accounts and Actions, *Qualitative Health Research*, **2**(4): 475–96.

Champion, R (1992) Professional Collaboration: The Lecturer Practitioner Role. In Bines M, Watson D (eds), *Developing Professional Education*, Milton Keynes: Open University.

Chandler, J (1991) Reforming Nurse Education 1: The Reorganisation of Nursing Knowledge, *Nurse Education Today*, **11**: 83–8.

Charlesworth, G, Kanneh, A and Masterson, N (1992) The Clinical Nurse Tutor Debate, *Nursing Times*, **88**(32): 40–1.

Cody, K (1994) Nursing Theory-guided Practice, What it Is and What it Is Not, *Nursing Science Quarterly*, **7**(4): 144–1.

Cohen, B (1985) Skills, Professional Education and the Disabling University, *Studies in Higher Education*, **10**(2): 175–85.

Cornes, D (1998) Some Thoughts on Nurse Education Service Partnerships, *Nurse Education Today*, **18**: 655–62.

Department of Health (1999) *Making a Difference: Strengthening the Nursing, Midwifery and Health Visiting Contribution to Health and Healthcare*, London: Stationery Office.

Doring, A, Bramwell, A and Bingham, B (1995) Staff Comfort/ Discomfort with Problem-based Learning: A Preliminary Study, *Nurse Education Today*, **15**(4): 263–6.

Elkan, R and Robinson, J (1993) Project 2000: The Gap Between Theory and Practice, *Nurse Education Today*, **13**: 295–8.

Eraut, M (1985) Knowledge Creation and Knowledge Use in Professional Contexts, *Studies in Higher Education*, **10**(2): 117–33.

Eraut, M (1994) *Developing Professional Knowledge and Competence*, London: Falmer Press.

Fay, P (1986) Contracting: A Collaborative Journal, *Journal of Nursing Staff Development*, **2**(4): 157–61.

Glen, S (1995) Towards a New Model of Nursing Education, *Nurse Education Today*, **15**: 90–5.

Glen, S and Clark, A (1999) Nursing Education: A Skill Mix for the Future, *Nurse Education Today*, **19**: 12–19.

Greenwood, J (1993) Reflective Practice, *Journal of Advanced Nursing*, **18**: 1183–7.

Lathlean, J (1992) The Contribution of Lecturer and Practitioners to Theory and Practice in Nursing, *Journal of Clinical Nursing*, **1**: 237–42.

Mackenzie, A E (1994) Bridging the Theory–Practice Gap: Learning from Experience, *Hong Kong Nursing Journal*, **65**(3).

Margetson, D (1994) Current Educational Reform and the Significance of Problem-based Learning, *Studies in Higher Education*, **19**(1): 5–19.

May, N, Vetch, L, McIntosh, J and Alexander, M (1997) *Preparation for Practice: Evaluation of Nurse and Midwife Education in Scotland, 1992 Programmes, Final Report*, Edinburgh: NBS.

Miller, A (1985) The Relationship between Nursing Theory and Nursing Practice, *Journal of Advanced Nursing*, **10**(5): 417–24.

Morse, J M (1996) Nursing Scholarship: Sense and Sensibility, *Nursing Inquirer*, **3**: 74–82.

National Health Service Executive (1998) Integrating Theory and Practice. A report commissioned by Chief Nursing Officer/ Director of Nursing

Prowse, M A (1996) Linking Knowledge and Practice through Teacher Led Placements for Students, *Nursing Standard*, **10**(33): 44–8.

Schön, D A (1983) *The Reflective Practitioner: How Professionals Think in Action*, Aldershot: Arena.

Smith, A and Russell, J (1991) Using Critical Learning Incidents in Nurse Education, *Nurse Education Today*, **11**: 284–91.

Squires, G (1990) *First Degree: The Undergraduate Curriculum*, Buckingham: Open University Press.

Townsend, J (1990) Problem-based Learning, *Nursing Times*, **86**(14): 61–2.

United Kingdom Central Council for Nursing, Midwifery and Health Visiting (1994) *A Statement of Strategic Intent*, London: UKCC.

United Kingdom Central Council for Nursing, Midwifery and Health Visiting (1999) *Fitness for Practice*, London: UKCC.

Varcoe, C, and Cresswell, S (1993) Hospitals and the Educational Institution: An Innovative Partnership for Nursing Speciality Education, *Journal of Continuing Education in Nursing*, **243**: 131–4.

Walsh, M (1997) Accountability and Intuition: Justifying Nurse Practice, *Nursing Standard*, **11**(23): 39–41.

Williams, L (1998) Study Matters, *Nursing Standard*, **12**(36): 4.

World Health Organisation (1993) *Increasing the Relevance of Education for Health Professionals: A Report of a WHO Study Group on Problem-solving Education for the Health Professions*, Geneva: WHO.

Index